Goodbye Alex

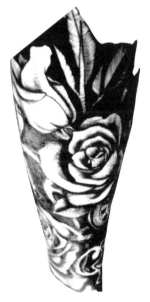

Len Kester

GOODBYE ALEX

Printed in the United States of America

This book is dedicated to both of my grandmothers. They each spent many, many hours, days, and weeks of their lives writing. They spent even more hours reading. Though neither of them published any of their works, I always saw dense, rich value in what I read from each of them. I don't know why they never published anything they wrote, but I'd like to think they would both be proud of me if they could see me now.

Brenda Gleave, or 'Nana' as we called her, was my maternal Grandmother. When I was young, I remember her listening to historians, archaeologists, and Biblical scholars. She put a hunger to learn inside me. She had been working on a fictional book set in medieval Scotland since before I can remember. She tinkered with this book, adding content, cutting content, and creating her own world. Without her influence and care, I wouldn't have chosen to write a book.

Elsie Lorraine Kester was my paternal Grandmother. She preferred for us to call her 'Maw-maw" though, so that's what we knew her by. She was the hardiest of humans, surviving breast cancer (twice). She wrote the most beautiful poems, and she adored frogs. I learned that her poems were a way for her to manage her own emotions, like a journal with a twist. I've learned that from her, and it's been a tremendously helpful practice through the years.

Nana, Maw-maw, I love and thank you both wherever you may be now.

Chapter 1

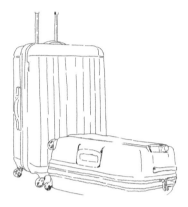

"Kinda like a cloud I was up way up in the sky, and I was feeling some feelings you wouldn't believe. Sometimes I don't believe them myself, and I decided I was never coming down..." Nine Inch Nails played across my headphones. I stared out the window of the heavy 747 and felt above it all. A silly grin spread across my face as I thought, "I'm actually moving across the country..." I proudly and naively wondered to myself if this is how success was always going to feel. I was elated.

"Ladies and Gentlemen, we're beginning our descent into San Diego now." Glued to my window, I saw the city come wholly into view through the sparse clouds. My eyes danced behind the window and caught the vast blue of the Pacific Ocean in the distance. My spine crawled with an instinctive shudder, and instead, I tried to focus on the landscape directly below.

As we descended, finer detail came into view. The cars crawled slowly through the gridded city streets, in and out of the long shadows of the tall palm trees. People scurried below like ants. I wondered where all the people were going. Weddings? Funerals? Business meetings? Court appearances? I made my guesses, but they all seemed meaningless from up here. The only thing that had any meaning was what existed in my own world and the things I was doing. But what meaning does that have compared to the backdrop of all the activity below me right now? Each person below probably felt the same way I did. I couldn't have the life I have without society, meaningless as it may feel to me. I could find appreciation in that, even if it was a bit paradoxical. The plane softly bumped on the runway and we started rapidly slowing.

My right leg was bouncing up and down as I waited my turn to get off the plane. I inhaled deeply and looked around, but nobody was moving. "Patience..." I tried reminding myself. I exhaled the breath that had been stuck in my chest for a minute now. I was so full of energy and growing more impatient by the moment, practically bursting.

I weaved my way through the crowd as quickly as I could before realizing I had no idea which way the exit was nor where I was heading. But slowing down wasn't an option and I needed to find an exit. I was so close I could almost taste it.

After what felt like endless corridors with endless people, I finally approached the exit next to my baggage claim. I sped up as much as I could without actually breaking into a jog and began fishing a cigarette from the pack in my pants pockets as I approached the exit.

The door didn't have a chance to close before that cigarette was lit. The first rush of nicotine in hours hit my veins and I could immediately feel my arms cool down and my head begin to clear up. I closed my eyes as I exhaled and then began to send out text updates.

"landed safely, will call asap love you!!!" I sent a text to my wife, Liz.

"plane landed, smoking outside baggage claim" I sent another text to my Uncle.

"where you at sucka???" Read a final text to my little brother, Donny.

I took another long drag from the lit cigarette, inhaled deeply, and just tried to enjoy the moment.

Bzzt bzzt. My phone vibrated in my hand. It was a reply text from my wife, and I couldn't help the big stupid grin that crept across my face as I read it. "good, send me pics!" it read.

Bzzt bzzt. Another vibration and another text. Bzzt bzzt. And another.

"standing in front of the baggage carousel, don't see you???" The text from Uncle William read.

"walking off the plane now," Donny's reply read.

I finished my precious nicotine stick as quickly as I could and headed back inside. I began to scan the crowd for Uncle William, but I wasn't seeing him anywhere.

"Lenny?" I heard my Uncle's voice ask from an ambiguous position in the distance behind me. I spun around excitedly and called back in our impromptu game of Marco Polo. "Uncle William?" I said in the direction I heard my name from. My eyes were still searching through the crowd when I heard, "Down here Lenny, ha-ha!" in Uncle William's voice and I looked about a foot lower than where I was scanning and saw my Uncle's face. The last time I saw him was when I was 16. I was only an inch or so taller than him then. But I was in my mid-twenties now and grown.

Uncle William stood at about 5'4" but was slender and fit. He had long, wavy hair that was dark and red. His face was long and flat, with a small nose and an ever-so-slightly-cleft chin. Pronounced dimples punctuated his smiles. I always thought he looked a lot like Willem Dafoe.

He wore some plain denim jeans with dress shoes and a button-up collared shirt that was a thatched red and white design. Business-casual.

I began laughing as soon as I saw him and ran in for a hug. "Wow! It's been forever! How've you been?" I asked.

"I didn't get any shorter, thanks for reminding me though! Ha-ha!" He replied in jest.

"Man... Heh... I'm... Ha-I'm s... sorry." I coughed out between stifled chuckles. I was trying to stop laughing, but it was funny, and this was a good moment. "I don't remember you being that short though." I quipped with a smirk.

"Oh, shut up." He said as he waved his hand dismissively at me and laughed. "Your little brother's plane landed a few moments ago too. You got your luggage yet?"

"Oh right!" The luggage carousel had started either while I was smoking or while I was looking for Uncle William, but I didn't notice the buzzer that announced it.

I watched luggage of all shapes and colors get carried around the conveyor belt and noticed my luggage just as it disappeared behind the black, plastic, flappy curtain. "Hmph," I thought, suddenly embarrassed. I froze up, trapped in my thoughts. How could I miss my baggage? In my mind, that was a failure and I had to make sure I corrected it. I scolded myself until I noticed my luggage come back around.

"Focus, Len..." I reminded myself silently, trying to escape my sudden and self-imposed mental prison. "You don't want people to think you're crazy." I noticed my luggage returning to me down the line a bit. "Nope, not again carousel!" I thought defiantly as I watched my luggage like a hawk this time.

"'Eeeeyyyyyy! What up you ol' basta'd!" I heard Donny's voice behind me as I was picking my luggage up.

Donny stood tall and proud at 5' 11". With short, dark brown hair, he pulled his lips together firmly and stood with his arms out.

"Donny? Oh my god..." Uncle William's mouth hung open in disbelief. "The last time I saw you, you were no bigger than my forearm and too small for your own diapers." Uncle William stepped over for a hug.

"Yeah, it's been a while man. How are you?" Donny's perfect dimples revealed themselves in a big smile.

"Hungry!" Uncle William gave an exaggerated expression, "I dunno about you guys, but I could go for a burrito. Get your stuff and let's go!"

"Oh, hell yeah!" I said. "I haven't eaten anything today, so my stomach is starting to digest itself."

"Yeah, sure. That sounds good." Donny also replied, his voice low and smooth as he went to grab his bags. I didn't remember him sounding so mature and refined from the last few months we spent apart.

Uncle William nodded with a smile, "Great. I know the BEST burrito place around the corner."

"You can ride shotgun, bud," I said and jumped straight in the car.

"Uh, yeah cool." Donny's voice sounded sarcastic. Almost like I had offended him somehow. Donny and Uncle William talked in the front while my thoughts lingered on that last interaction. I didn't understand how to process his response.

In the back seat, my inner thoughts went full steam ahead. I'd silently hoped the little things I did would show Donny I cared about him, even if we hadn't seen much of each other over the last 10 years since I went to college and got married. I could tell him that I care, but I figured showing it would go a lot further. Donny and I had to learn whom each other had become over the last 10 years and re-establish our relationship as brothers. I was excited and curious to see what he would do as he grew into adulthood.

I shook my head and stepped out of the car when we arrived. We walked in, placed our orders, and found an empty table to sit at. I was the last to order, so I poured my horchata from the drink machine and joined Uncle William and Donny at the table they chose.

"Mmmmmmm..." I said with surprise as I took my first gulp of the horchata.

"Have you never had an horchata before?" Uncle William asked me.

"Nope. First one. I've been missing out." I replied with a goofy grin.

Uncle William shook his head. "My god you boys have been living under a rock."

"I know what an horchata is." Donny said.

"Okay, well only you have been living under a rock, Lenny." Uncle William said.

"Not anymore. I know what an horchata is now, so I can live with the rest of you cool kids." I said in half-jest and half-annoyance but trying to keep it light. I could feel some uneasiness well up inside and didn't understand why.

"Nope, you still live under a rock, ha-ha!" Donny said. I found it uncomfortable, but I laughed it off. Donny laughed, then Uncle William laughed.

"Ok good, I guess I handled that the right way?" I thought to myself, feeling the lightness in the air return and replace my confusion.

We finished our meals and went back to Uncle William's house. As we pulled up, I noticed the windows were open. I had been out to Uncle William's house once before when I was 16, and I distinctly remember the windows always being open and the house always feeling comfortable. That was comforting to see no change there.

"Ok, boys." Uncle William addressed us both as we walked in the front door, "I've got a blow-up mattress in the back office, and a couch in the living room." He pointed around the small house as he spoke and walked, "There are sheets and pillows in this closet here." He stopped and turned to face us, "I expect you both to fold your sheets every morning and put them back into the closet. If you have the couch, please fluff it back up to make it not look like it has been slept on all night. If you have the air mattress, please deflate it, and put it away every morning." Uncle William's demeanor was suddenly all business, and I was a little jarred by the sudden change.

Did I do something for him to start acting this way? Was it something I said at the airport or at the restaurant? I froze up insecurely and my brain went racing with thoughts again.

I realized I was frozen and had to respond, "Absolutely." I said blindly, realizing I may have missed a few words from him just then, "I'll be sure to take care of my stuff each day. Thanks for letting us both stay here, Uncle William." I wanted to be sure I thanked him. This was a nice thing he was doing for us both. Not overstaying my welcome was something I was thinking about and gauging already, and I felt like it started here and now by being thankful and showing respect.

I offered to take the air mattress first. Uncle William dismissed us, and I texted Liz as I went back to my room.

"Hey you, we made it to Uncle William's house. Getting settled now. I'll call as soon as I can get some time alone." I hit the send button.

Once I finished texting Liz, I started looking for a place to keep my luggage. I scanned the room, found a place to plug my phone charger in, put my toothbrush and toothpaste into the bathroom, and grabbed an empty trash bag to keep my dirty clothes in.

Uncle William popped his head in the room just then, "Hey, what're you doing up here? Haven't you noticed we're downstairs? You coming?" His voice dripped with impatience.

"What? No, I didn't know you guys were downstairs nor that I had to be there. I was just putting my stuff up. I'll be down momentarily." I defended myself, still unsure why I was being summoned. I hated being rushed.

Uncle William turned and waved for me to follow him. So, I reluctantly did. We walked through the single-story home, out the back door, and down the wooden steps into his tiny backyard. Once I got to the bottom of the steps, I noticed Donny sitting at a dimly lit glass table out on the lawn and holding a joint up for me. It was nighttime now, so only the glow of a single candle and the moonlight highlighted their faces.

"It's your hit, man." Donny strained, holding a lungful in.

I immediately smiled and got excited. I don't mean only about smoking weed together, though that was certainly part of it. But I was thinking of a ton of other things that we could find comradery in now that he was older and more mature. We could go into business together if we wanted to. How cool would that be? We could talk about life experiences and help each other navigate life's problems now. The age difference between us suddenly mattered significantly less, and that felt awesome. Changing all those baby diapers was paying off in ways I'd never imagined.

I walked up and grabbed the joint from Donny and took a big drag. "Wow, I haven't had brick weed in a long time." I said, also with a lungful. The taste reminded me of my teenage years, scraping together $10 for a dime bag. After a moment of nostalgia, I passed the joint to Uncle William and exhaled.

"You know they have way better shit out there now, right old man?" Donny said to Uncle William with a laugh.

"Yeah, yeah, yeah..." Uncle William replied, "I'm old-fashioned. I just don't see the need to smoke that weed. I mean, you only get so high, right? Seems like a waste of money to me."

I displayed my best, "Whatever floats your boat" face and sat down across the table from Uncle William.

"So why didn't your twin come with you?" Uncle William inhaled and passed the joint to Donny.

"Alex is too busy being lazy, I guess," Donny replied critically, taking the joint. "He's got a bunch of junkie friends he doesn't want to leave up there in Indiana." He took a long drag and passed the joint to me.

I took the joint and stared at it. My thoughts were on Alex now though. Junkie friends? What happened to my little Alex?

"GWAHAHA!" baby Alex laughed hysterically. He had made a huge mess with his spaghetti, and it was all over the highchair, the wall, the table, the floor, and his face. Donny sat across the table in another highchair and stared at Alex in wonder. Donny was much cleaner, only having a little bit of spaghetti on one hand and a little bit on his face. Mom handed me a wet washcloth.

I wiped his face and hands, and he immediately slapped a pile of spaghetti sauce and cut-up noodle bits in front of him, which now decorated my shirt and glasses. Things seemed so much simpler then.

I smiled in reaction to the memory but had accidentally let the joint go out.

"Party foul!" Donny pointed at me and laughed. He still had the same laugh as he did on the night of flying spaghetti nearly 19 years ago.

"Yeah sorry, got lost in thought for a moment there." I chuckled, grabbed the lighter that Uncle William slid across the table to me, and held the joint between my lips, "We gotta get Alex out of Indiana. That place is a sucking pit of despair." I shook my head lightly and paused to light the joint between my lips and inhaled deeply, "If he's in with a bad group of friends, that's not gonna go well for him."

Uncle William nodded, "Yep," he responded emphatically, "That's why I was really hoping he would come down here with you, Donny. I want you guys to take over my business eventually. I'm getting too old for this shit." He chuckled.

"Yeah, if he wants to hang out with his loser friends and go nowhere, that's his choice I guess." Donny replied, taking the joint from Uncle William. "He doesn't know what he wants."

Uncle William shook his head, "That's sad, but all I can do is provide the opportunity."

Donny took another large drag and passed the joint to me, which was now getting awfully short to comfortably hold. "You have anything I could use for a roach clip, Uncle William?" I asked, taking what was left of the joint carefully between my thumb and forefinger.

"Don't be a bitch," Donny said, laughing.

Uncle William laughed, "Yeah I've got some hemostat clamps in the shed there." He pointed under the deck.

As I walked to go look for the clamps, my thoughts gravitated back to Alex.

"I wanna drive a big truck and marry an ugly big truck wife when I grow up!" 6-year-old Alex said.

"What?" I replied, confused. I had hoped I didn't hear him right.

"Yeah! I wanna drive a big truck and marry an ugly big truck wife!"

He repeated with the most innocent smile on his face and giggled.

I laughed it off, thinking he was being funny and didn't mean what he said, "Is that right?" I asked. "Well, if that's what you really want to do, you can I guess," I reassured him and questioned my sanity.

"No, I wanna be like you. I wanna be bad like you and I'm gonna die when I'm 26," he replied with that same innocent grin still plastered across his face.

Struck by his comment, I recoiled, "Aw, hey buddy... don't say that. Why would you say that? You know I'm not trying to be bad, right?" My own 16-year-old brain struggled to find words that stood up to any semblance of reason. Saddened and confused, I continued, "Mom and Dad just don't understand why I want to do the things I do."

I found the hemostat clamps in the shed and headed back out to the table. I fixed what was left of the joint into the clamps, grabbed Uncle William's lighter, and lit it again as I sat down. "You know..." I said with a lungful, "It would have been awesome if Alex had come out here," I exhaled, "But I still plan on making the most of my opportunity here. Maybe we can still provide him with an opportunity that looks appealing to him in the future." I passed the clamps to Uncle William.

Uncle William waved a hand to let me know he didn't want it, "No thanks, it's almost bedtime for me anyway. Donny," he continued, addressing my brother, "Are you ready to get to work tomorrow? I've got a full day planned for us." He started grinning and laughing.

"Fo' sho'" Donny replied positively. "I'll go get the couch ready and try to catch some sleep."

"Yeah, I've got work in the morning, too. I'd like to be rested for my first day there," I said while offering the joint to Donny, but he refused as well. "Oh, don't be a bitch, Donny." I said, returning the joke from earlier. It got no response from either of them, so I just sat in awkward silence and puffed the rest of the joint. Uncle William and Donny got up and went upstairs to turn in for the night.

I sat at the table in the yard and smoked a couple cigarettes, lost in thought. Something felt weird and not right. Premonitions of abstract failure pooled up inside, and I wasn't sure why. I tried to sort it out but got tired and decided to head to bed. "Hhhhnnnn..." I groaned, shook my head, and put my cigarette out. I concluded in my mind that I was just dealing with a little bit of anxiety and just needed to go to bed and let the emotion come and go on its own.

Chapter 2

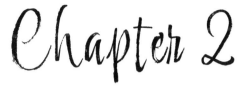

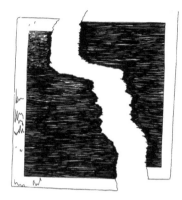

I blinked awake for the third time and looked at my phone. 4:30 AM. "Hmph," I thought out loud. "Don't do this now..." I was both nervous and excited at the same time about my first day of work out here in San Diego. I just wanted to get started, so that I could get it over with faster.

I tossed and turned for the next several minutes, unable to shut my brain off. I played through different scenarios of my first day at work, thinking about all the typical challenges we faced in customer-facing computer repair and how to act like a professional and not 'the new guy'.

I decided to get up when I heard Uncle William get up and start a shower. "Coffee time..." My brain was now finally singular in its focus and began folding the sheets and blankets, deflating the air mattress, and putting Uncle William's office back together. After I was done, I headed toward the door. I stopped just short of the closed office door and turned to look at the room. It looked just like it did when I found it, except for my bags in the corner. I made sure to leave nothing on his desk where my phone had been charging. I smiled in approval and turned to head out the door with the sheets under my arm.

I put the sheets in the closet on my way to the kitchen and started making coffee. I looked for the coffee grinder for a couple minutes before realizing the coffee was pre-ground. Rubbing my eye, I searched around the kitchen until I found the filters and put it all together on the coffee cart. I eagerly punched the 'on' button and stared at the coffee machine as though I could simply will it to go faster.

"Why you staring at the coffee machine in your pajamas, Len?" Donny let out a stifled laugh and walked past me to fill a glass with water at the sink.

"Yeah, I'm still waking up. I need this coffee to hurry or for the shower to free up." I responded automatically and matter-of-factly, not awake yet.

Donny shook his head, "Goofy-ass..."

I looked into the living room and the couch still had his sheets on it, "Don't forget to take care of your bedding stuff." I said without a pause for thought.

Just then, I heard the bathroom door open. "Well good morning boys."

"Morning," I responded dryly.

"Sup old man?" Donny said energetically.

"What's your problem, Len?" Uncle William asked, combing his still-wet hair.

"Problem? No problem. I'm just not awake yet." I responded, confused why he thought I had a problem at all.

"Well, get on it because you have your first day of work today and you don't need to be fucking around." Uncle William pointed his hairbrush at me.

I felt the tingling warmth of anger starting at the back of my skull. "Yeah, I'm aware." I said defensively. I knew I needed to manage that and not respond emotionally, but he was making things very difficult. I denied my mouth the approval to say the rest of the words that were dying to fall out of it. "After a shower and some coffee, I'll be fine." I assured him.

"Dibs on the shower! Hahahaha!" Donny said and ran into the bathroom and locked the door.

I inhaled deeply and turned back to watch the coffee pot. Once the coffee was finished, I poured a cup and stepped out to the back patio for a smoke while I drank some coffee and woke up.

I didn't have to be at work until 10AM, and it was only 8AM. I had plenty of time, so I didn't stress about the shower. I just took my time to enjoy the coffee and cigarettes as I woke up and got ready for work.

"Alright, I'll be back to pick you up at 6PM when your shift ends. I hope you have a good day." Uncle William said through the driver's window as he dropped me off for work.

"Yep, that's perfect. Thank you, Uncle William, I really appreciate the ride. Hope you guys have a good day too!" I smiled and double-tapped the roof of the car before turning to head inside. Clad in my iconic short-sleeved white button-up dress shirt, black clip-on tie, black dress slacks, white high-top socks, and black high-gloss Oxford shoes, I marched confidently into the Best Buy before me.

As was my ritual back home, I walked behind the Geek Squad precinct and clocked in at the agent terminal.

As soon as I clocked in, another agent came up behind me, "Oh you must be Len!" she exclaimed excitedly. A shorter woman with long red hair in a ponytail was standing in front of me reaching her hand out for a shake. "I'm Becca!"

I smiled and returned the handshake. "That's right, I'm the new guy around here!" I responded with a laugh.

With a shake and a nod, Becca continued, "The others are in the break room right now, but they should be out here in a minute. You want me to show you what we have on the bench?"

Straight to work. I liked Becca already. "Absolutely! Point me to the problems so I can find some solutions." I responded with a smile.

"Are you Len?" A new, deep voice behind me said. Three other agents walked into the precinct behind us.

I turned around and nodded with a smile, "That's me!" I reached out my hand in the direction of the voice.

"I'm Brian," The deep voice said. Brian stood tall, towering over me. I thought I was a tall guy at 6'1". He was skinny, like me. He had medium length dirty blonde hair, and wore thick glasses, like me. Even though his voice was low and deep, he had a disposition about him that made him seem like one of the kindest, most gentle people I would ever meet. Brian shook my outstretched hand and continued, "This is Mauricio," he pointed to his left.

"Sup." Mauricio said, keeping one hand in his pocket and the other holding a Sprite. He had wavy jet-black hair and dark olive toned skin, indicative of his Latin lineage.

Brian pointed at the third agent, "And this," he continued, "is Nate."

Nate stepped forward to offer a handshake with an excited smile, "What's up? What're you into? You play any video games or board games?" Nate was speaking my language. He was the shortest of the bunch, standing lower than Becca and always slightly hunching his shoulders. He had longer wavy brown hair and his right eye was always extremely blood-shot.

I could feel my eyebrows raise with anticipation and excitement, "Oh yeah, my wife and I play WoW. That's our main thing, but we play a lot of different video games together. We do that instead of watching TV shows."

"What about snorkeling? You ever been snorkeling?" His words were still hurried and excited.

"Nope! Never been snorkeling. In Mississippi, all we have are swamps. Not snorkel-friendly at all." I joked with a laugh behind the words.

Nate laughed genuinely in return, "Well I know some amazing places to snorkel around here if you ever want to come with me someday."

"Oh boy, he's already going for the snorkel." Mauricio commented and moved to one of the PCs on the tech bench and got to work, silently sipping on his Sprite.

"Nate loves snorkeling, and you would be his friend forever if you ever went with him." Brian said with his deep and friendly voice. The more that Brian talked, the more I identified with his personality.

"I might have to take you up on that sometime, Nate." I responded. "Becca was just showing me which PCs still have unresolved issues back here, so I'm going to get busy. It's great meeting everyone!"

The rest of my shift was just the same as it would have been back in Mississippi. I spent my time talking to clients, fixing the myriad of Windows issues on our tech bench, and cataloguing everything in the system. It was satisfying to be the new guy and not need any training. In fact, I was helping some of my new co-workers with some unique issues they ran across. The over-achiever in me was placated.

Uncle William picked me up promptly at 6PM, after my first shift was over. The ride home was quiet, other than a short discussion about what to have for dinner. I smoked a cigarette and watched the city move past me through the open window of the backseat, reflecting on my day silently. I was tired, but otherwise in a good mood that my first day had gone well.

Back at the table in Uncle William's back yard, I unwrapped my first fish taco that we got on the way home, "So what did you guys do today?" I asked as I slathered hot sauce onto the taco.

"We helped Frank. Tell him about Frank, Donny." Uncle William said and took a bite of his own taco.

"It's super sad about Frank." Donny started before taking a small bite and continuing to talk, "He used to be a millionaire, but something happened like 10 years ago that made him like, I dunno retarded? Is that right?" Donny finished chewing.

Uncle William gulped a bite down, "Frank is clinically retarded now, yeah. And my business is taking care of people like Frank who need assistance in their daily lives. Over 10 years ago now, Frank suffered an accident on-site at his construction business that he owned. His whole world fell apart in 30 seconds. And so, we take him to the store, manage his budget, oversee his in-home care, and make sure his family doesn't steal his fortune."

Still chewing, I mused on Frank's misfortune and regarded my own health. It both terrified me that someone could lose their faculties like that yet also made me extremely thankful for my own health. "Man..." my eyebrows scrunched up with empathy, "That's a rough lot in life."

Uncle William shrugged, swallowed, and set his empty taco wrapper on the table, "What can you do but be helpful?"

"Are all of the clients disabled like Frank?" Donny asked, balling up his taco wrapper and fiddling with the paper ball.

"Yep, sure are. All of them in some way need help and have been granted government assistance. If they don't qualify for government assistance, I can't help them. My business depends on that government assistance. We've got a court appearance to make tomorrow so we can vouch for continued support for another one of my clients." Uncle William said.

The table now had empty taco wrappers strewn about and our bellies were full. "What about your day, Lenny?" Uncle William asked as he started rolling a joint.

"It was a good day." I responded, full of good energy. "I met all my new co-workers, which is rare that all five of us agents were there at once. I resolved 3 different PCs issues today, one of which had been there for 7 days now with no resolution. It felt good to solve that one. I guess the customer put a bunch of restrictions on what we were allowed to do to fix the issue, and so I got into the registry and made manual edits..."

Uncle William put his hand up, stopping me. "Ok, ok, you lost me there. Keep it simple."

"Oh, sorry. Yeah, good day." I said tersely, both frustrated that I was interrupted and disappointed that he seemed to not care. I became aware that my tone of voice probably showed my emotions more than I wanted.

Uncle William looked at me blankly for a moment in awkward silence, then lit the joint. "In any case, we've got a long day ahead of us tomorrow, Donny."

"Yeah, I'm not excited about being in a courtroom, but let's go!" Donny's tone was avid.

I lurched my shoulders in discomfort, "Court doesn't sound great at all. I'll take my computer problems over all that any day."

"I can understand the court system." Uncle William paused to hit the joint, "I can't understand these damn computers." He squinted, speaking softly with full lungs.

Donny reached out to take the joint Uncle William was holding out with a snorting chuckle, "Get with the times, old man!" He was laughing too hard to hit the joint.

"Puff, puff, pass, duuuude!" Uncle William waggled a finger at Donny, drawing the last word out emphatically and laughing.

I wondered why Uncle William seemed more jovial toward Donny and I got lost in my thoughts. "Oh, my bad!" I said, realizing that Donny was passing me the joint. I took it and hit it quickly, keeping it moving through the rotation quickly.

Uncle William carefully took the joint I handed him and puffed, "So..." He puffed again, keeping the joint to his lips as he spoke, "The next day off we all have," he puffed again, "I want to take you boys to Black Bleach." With a final puff, he handed the joint to Donny. "Have you ever been to a nude beach, Donny?"

"Fuck yeah! Let's go to the nude beach!" Donny almost bounced up and down in his chair with laughter and excitement as he took the joint.

"Easy there, killer." I raised one eyebrow in jest, making a silly face as I grabbed the joint from him. "The nude beach probably isn't the experience you have pictured in your mind's eye right now." I took a big drag from the joint, trying to one-up Donny. It burned until I couldn't help a coughing fit. Self-aware, I was laughing and coughing as I tried passing the joint to Uncle William.

Uncle William held up his hand, "No thanks, it's too short." He continued, "The nude beach is..." He paused, "...an experience. Teh-heh-heh-heh!" He put extra emphasis on the word 'experience' and pressed his tongue against the back of his teeth and laughed sinisterly in a high pitch.

I laughed too, feeling good that I was on the inside of a joke instead of the brunt of it. I handed the remainder of the joint to Donny, "Who knows? You might get lucky."

Donny took the joint, "I'd really be happy just going to any beach. The riverbank in Memphis isn't cool unless you like mud." He joked and puffed on the stub of a joint between his fingers before offering it to me.

I waved a hand, "No thanks bud, I'm good for now. It really is too short to hold comfortably."

Donny mocked, his voice full of sarcasm, "Don't be a bitch, Donny."

I couldn't help a laugh, and the whole table erupted in laughter.

"Well," I said inhaling deeply and standing up, "I need to go get more cigarettes. I'm out and I need some nicotine."

Uncle William immediately offered me one of his cigarettes, "Here, have one of mine. You need to be saving your money."

I must have looked as confused as I was. "What? Naw it's all good. I don't want to use your supply of cigarettes. You smoke those fancy, expensive American Spirits. I just buy the cheap Camels. I'll make an effort to smoke less though, if that'll make you feel more comfortable about me hemorrhaging money." I said sincerely, trying to manage that whole 'overstaying-my-welcome' thing.

"Whatever." He replied quickly, seeming irritated.

Still confused, I shook it off and said, "I'm just going to walk to the gas station around the corner. I'll be back in a minute. Does anyone need anything while I'm making the trip there?"

"No, save your money, Lenny." Uncle William was unmistakably irritated now.

The store was only a 5-minute walk, but it went so fast because I was wrapped up in my thoughts trying to analyze what just occurred before I went to get cigarettes. I looked down at the ground in front of me as I walked. Growing up in Memphis as a white boy, I learned to keep my head down and mind my own business and not look curious.

I wondered if maybe he thought I was being sarcastic with him. Maybe he just wants me to try his cigarettes? Maybe he's just worried that I'll mismanage my finances and he'll have to put up with me for longer? But what's so bad about me? Is there something I'm doing wrong? What is he not seeing that he's expecting to see?

I entered the store and lifted my head from gazing at the ground, "Hey, yeah, let me get..." I said. I thought about buying 5 packs of cigarettes so I'd have plenty for the week, but thought I'd buy less to help placate Uncle William's concerns, hoping that would mean something to him. "...2 packs of Camel Wides in the box, please."

"Thanks," I said as the cashier handed me the receipt and my cigarettes. I put one pack into my pocket and flipped the other one upside down and started slapping it against the palm of my hand. I opened the fresh pack of smokes, put one in my lips, and lit it.

"Ahhh," I thought to myself as I inhaled fresh nicotine and carcinogens. It wasn't enough to pull my mind away from the interaction with Uncle William though, and I continued to stress over it on my way back to Uncle William's house.

When I got back to Uncle William's house, he and Donny were on the couch looking at a box of old photos. I wanted to avoid Uncle William to prevent me saying anything that might get on his nerves or cause another awkward interaction, so I headed back to the office to get my bedding setup for the night.

"Hey, where are you headed in such a hurry?" Uncle William asked, "Don't you want to come see some of these photos?"

I groaned internally but tried to respond amicably. I didn't want to respond negatively and piss him off any more. "Sure, let me just get my bed s-"

Uncle William interrupted, "You've got time. We're doing this now. Come on over." He patted the couch and as he looked at me, I swear I could feel a challenge in his eye to defy him. Why was this weirdness between us?

Donny looked at Uncle William ignorantly, then me.

I hated the way he interrupted me and challenged wills the way he did. I couldn't let my irritation show though. That wouldn't make things any better. "Alrighty then." I said in defeat, certain that my irritation was oozing out of the seams anyway. I didn't want Uncle William to ask me what my problem was, because I might have been blatantly honest with him in that moment. That had nuclear potential, and I knew it.

I sat down next to Donny, getting the pictures after he saw them. I took a small stack of pictures that they had already gone through while I was walking and began to flip through them to catch up.

I picked up a picture of Uncle William and became raptured by a memory I had almost completely forgotten about.

Uncle William and I were sitting on his couch in his old house. He handed me a picture and I took it. It was a picture of a naked guy from the chest down, no face. I was suddenly overwhelmingly uncomfortable and confused. I thought we were going to be looking at old photos of him and mom. I wasn't really sure how to react. "Uh... oh..." I stammered. I needed an exit from this, and fast.

"That's me." Uncle William said with a weird grin.

Houston, we have a problem. "What? Aww, no, I don't want to see this, man. You're my Uncle." I dropped the photo on the couch and got up, uneasy and confused.

"Good, I, uh, wanted to make sure you didn't have a thing for me..." Uncle William said sheepishly in response.

I snapped out of the memory, retaining all the uneasiness I found there. I closed my eyes and breathed very slowly. What the hell was I supposed to do with this memory? I needed a cigarette.

"That was cool," I commented after we were finished looking through the photo album. "I am going to go smoke and then get my bed setup."

"I'll go with." Donny said, "I need a smoke, too."

"Looks like I'm going downstairs for another smoke as well." Uncle William said.

I hadn't had the time alone that I needed to quell the vortex of thoughts in my mind. I felt like I was being pressured into an uncomfortable and potentially destructive interaction but didn't know how to respond. I felt extremely uneasy after remembering that interaction.

I finally made it to my room after a couple cigarettes and called Liz.

"Hey!" my wife's voice brought a wave of calm over me.

"Hey you!" I replied excitedly.

"How's it going out in sunny California?" She asked.

My head bounced back and forth, "Things are..." I paused for thought, "... weird."

"Just think about how much better it will be once I move out there too." She reassured me.

I smiled, "Yeah, I can't wait for that. That seems so far away, but you're right. I need to just stay focused on the goal of getting us moved out here and not get caught up in the little things."

"Good. Have you seen any places you want to start looking at?" She asked.

"I have!" I replied excitedly, "There's a couple places I saw on my way in to work today that I'd like to find out more about. I saved the numbers in my phone to call later. I'll probably save numbers until my next day off then make a bunch of calls all at once."

"Ohh, send me pictures when you go!" Her excitement was contagious, and it was pulling me into a better place, emotionally.

"Absolutely! If you want, we can figure out how to do a video call and I can take you, like, on a virtual tour with me when I go!" I was proud of that idea, and it had just hit me.

"Ohh yeah, I forgot our new phones have video now." She remembered.

"Yeah, I'll figure that out soon. It shouldn't be too hard. How was your day?" I asked, already feeling less anxious.

"I think I'm getting the hang of this new manager role. I did my first interview today and I think I'm going to hire them." She stated proudly.

"Oooohhhhh," I did my best to exaggerate a sense of grandeur, "Doing interviews already? What's next, world domination?" I stifled a laugh.

"Hahaha, yes, Pinky, tomorrow we try to take over the world!" She feigned her best evil Brain voice.

My face almost hurt from all the smiling I was doing, "Well, I think I'm going to get ready for bed, babe. I'm tired."

"Okay, I miss you!" She said sweetly.

"I miss you too, baby. Looking forward to getting you out here with me!" I said, feeling the distance between us. I wanted to give her a hug.

"Mmmmyeeeeessssssss..." I could imagine her fingers steepled as she said that in her evil Brain voice again.

"Good night my baby! I love you!" I said, feeling all the love in that moment.

"Good night!"

Chapter 3

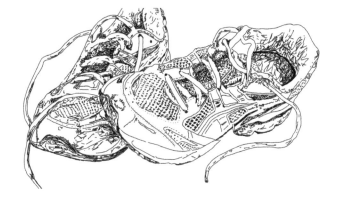

I sat across the table from Uncle William, eyes glossing over from the intense lecture I was receiving. "I thought you'd be a man." Uncle William said frustrated, "You haven't offered to pay rent, you haven't offered to contribute to the weed pool, and you haven't paid me back for any of my cigarettes you've smoked." He squinted his eyes and frowned in judgement.

My eyebrows scrunched up in confusion and I leaned forward over the table, "I thought we agreed that this would be rent free because I'm still paying bills back home? Besides, anytime I mention spending money you get shitty with me." I couldn't help the frustration in my tone. "What do you want? You tell me how you want to see me spending my money then. You give me a dollar-for-dollar breakdown of how you would be happy with how I spend my money, ok?" I could feel myself starting to not care about any consequences. Fuck it, here goes.

I gave in to the emotions and my voice started cracking with stress, "I offered to buy weed and you wouldn't let me. Or do you not remember that day? I can't keep up with you dude. I think you're just going to be mad at me no matter what I do, so fuck it." I was trying not to raise my voice, but the emotional well inside was building too much pressure.

"This isn't working. You're going to have to find your own way to work now. I can't keep driving you around." He loathed.

"Yeah, whatever." I scowled. "I offered to pay for gas too, but you said no. But I guess I'm going to hear how disappointed you are in me for not paying for the gas anyway, right?"

"Alright, alri-" He started.

"No, what do you want from me?" Upset, I interrupted him for a change, "I'm doing my dead-level best to make this work, but I can't fight against you the whole time." Exasperated, I paused.

"Look, maybe you should consider going back home." He said calmly.

I shook my head emphatically, "That's not an option, and you know it. I came out here with the goal of moving my family here. I can't just put it down and give up on it like that. I'm due for a raise at work in a couple weeks. I'm serious about this and I'm making real progress. As soon as I get that raise, I should be able to get my own place," I reasoned. "I'm close."

Uncle William raised his eyebrows in disbelief and steepled his fingers, "Bless your heart." He patronized.

Why was he being an ass? I could feel my emotions escalating even further. "Do you remember showing me that nude pic on your couch when I was out here as a teenager? What the hell was that all about?" Shiiiiiit... why did I say that?

"What? No, I don't remember that." He protested, a look of disgust spreading across his face.

Overcome with frustration in the moment, my face contorted "Well, it happened. You told me it was you." Where the hell was I going with this? Did I really expect him to admit to it? I had to get control of my emotions. "Anyway, what the fuck ever man. I can't tell why, but from my perspective it looks to me like you're just going to be shitty with me no matter what I do, so why even try?" I ended the question with my arms in the air.

"That's just sad." He replied, shaking his head slowly, fingers still steepled.

"Fuckin' tell me about it." I responded sarcastically and lit a cigarette. As I calmed down, I wondered if he was trying to push my buttons to incite an emotional response. If so, I was playing right into it. No matter what, I had to calm down. Frustration was at an 11. "I'm going for a run." I said decidedly.

He un-steepled his fingers to look at his watch, "At 9PM?" He questioned.

"Yup." I replied tersely, put my cigarette out, and walked off.

I went to my room and grabbed my running clothes and shoes. As I picked up my running shoes, faded and worn, I thought about my victories I had while wearing them.

270 lbs. of disappointment weighed me down and I hated myself for it. I woke up at 3AM, put my brand-new running shoes on and ran my first of many miles in them. Well, if I'm honest I only jogged one-fourth of that mile that first day and walked the rest, completely out of breath. By the end of the second week, I could jog the entire mile. And by the end of the first month, I could run an 8-minute-mile. Fueled by the discontent I felt for myself, I lost 75 lbs. over those 3 months of running. Nothing helped my confidence and attitude like running did, and I accomplished all of it while wearing these shoes.

Holding my pair of shoes there in Uncle William's office, I found some respect for myself and a way to calm down. I had plateaued in weight but running had become cathartic. I'd always feel better after a run. It had become less about the weight loss and more about the emotional regulation by now.

I put my running outfit on, squeezed my headphones in, cranked up some Juno Reactor as loud as it would go and headed out for a run.

When I got back, I felt so much better. I had come to the decision to get a bus pass and use the public transport system to get to work. That seemed like an easy and obvious solution once I had calmed down.

That next weekend, on my next day off, I wanted to go to the beach with Donny. We grabbed our towels, threw on some flip-flops and board shorts, and boarded the bus to the beach.

I scratched my head, and smoothed out my hair after I sat down next to Donny on the bus. "Man, what do you think Uncle William's problem with me is? I'm really trying to figure out what, if anything, I've done wrong." I mused.

Donny shrugged, "I dunno... He's been fine to me."

"Have you seen the way he acts toward me though? Am I losing my mind, or does he seem to always get really... pissy with me?" I asked sincerely.

"Yeah, I have seen him act kinda like an ass to you a couple of times." Donny admitted.

I shook my head in confusion, "He cornered me the other night when you were helping Tom chop wood. Said things weren't working and he wasn't going to be giving me a ride to work anymore. That's his prerogative, but I just don't understand what I did to deserve that. The bus made me over an hour late 2 days last week, and over 3 hours late on a third day. I'm going to have to walk 8 miles to work to guarantee I'll be there on time."

Donny shrugged again, "That sucks. Just try not to let him get at you. He's a lonely old man."

I ran my fingers through my short hair, "I guess... I just... I wish I understood what was happening. I don't know if I can achieve my goal in this situation with him."

Donny looked at me sideways, "What goal?"

Surprised, I blinked, "I'm trying to move out here with Liz, bud." I said. I thought he knew what I was doing out here. "What did you think I was doing?"

Donny looked thoughtful for a minute, "I dunno, hangin' out because I'm here?"

I shook my head, "No, I'm trying to move out here. I'm a tech guy. All the good tech jobs are out here in California, not in Mississippi. There's no opportunity for me there unless I want to be stuck in basic computer repair for the rest of my life, which I most definitely do not want."

Donny cocked his head, "I guess that makes sense."

I wondered how I could have been so misunderstood. Did Uncle William also think I was 'just hangin' out' too? That would explain a lot, but it made me feel like I wasn't being taken seriously. I had announced my plans to move here openly, and I thought everyone around me understood that. Apparently not...

We had arrived at the beach and laid our towels out on the sand. I was ok laying on my beach towel and not going into the water. In fact, I hated the idea of being in the water when I couldn't see the bottom.

"Oh, don't be a bitch, Len, C'mon!" Donny urged me to come swimming in the ocean with him.

I sat down on my towel and looked up at him, "I'll stay here and guard the towels, haha." I joked, hoping he'd give up on it.

"Man..." he sighed and gave me a disappointed look.

"I'm sorry bubba, but I just do not want to get in the water." I kept looking at him and started feeling guilty. "Oh my god, alright let's go. But I'm only going up to my ankles. I'm not going out any further than that."

Donny's disappointment transmuted into excitement, "Awww, yeah!" He smiled and fist-pumped into the air.

We waded out and I stopped where I was comfortable stopping, "So you're leaving next week, yeah?" I asked.

Donny waded out a little further, up to his knees and turned around, "Yeah."

I could feel the seaweed wrapping around the top of my feet and fought the shudders. "So, what're you thinking? About working for Uncle William?" I asked, keeping my eyes down at my feet.

Donny inhaled deeply, "Oh I dunno... Samuel wants me to come work for him at the hydro shop in Memphis. I'm thinking about doing that instead."

I froze instantly. Samuel... that name bounced violently around inside my skull, hitting all the alarms on its way around.

I was just waking up. I was groggy as we'd smoked some weed and did some drinking the night before. Samuel and I had passed out in my bed. But something was off... what was it? What was happening right now? Coming to, I could hear a whimpering voice, "Please... please let me do this... give me a sign..." But I was frozen in panic. I realized that I had an erection and Samuel was fondling me. I didn't want this. I didn't want this at all. Why did I have an erection? I wanted to implode out of existence.

I pretended to be asleep hoping the moment would just go away and not happen. Maybe if I gave him no sign of interest, he would get the hint. He didn't. I stayed frozen, not sure what to do, while he performed oral sex on me. An orgasm should feel good, but I just wanted to cry. This is not how I pictured my first sexual experience. I thought I did something that gave him the wrong idea, and whatever had happened was my fault somehow. I pretended to be asleep for another few minutes before getting up and pretending that it never happened.

Some seaweed wrapped itself around my ankle, pulling me from my memory and I jumped. "Nope nope nope!" I exclaimed as I ran out of the water. "Don't like that seaweed at all. I'm going back to my towel, bubba." I calmed myself, more startled by the memory than the seaweed, but totally using the seaweed as my escape. I reminded myself to do the same thing I always did whenever I thought about that day, just try to ignore it. I laid out on my towel and decided to close my eyes and focus on the warmth of the sun.

"Uuughhhgh..." I groaned the next morning. I felt horrible. My body ached, I felt slightly sick to my stomach, had a terrible headache, and my skin was on fire. I wasn't about to call out of work though. I took a cold shower and carefully put my running clothes on. It felt like I was wearing sandpaper. I walked to work and changed in the bathroom before clocking in and getting to work.

"Woah Len, you look like hell. Are you alright?" Brian asked me.

"Man, I feel like shit. I spent the day at the beach yesterday and got pretty sunburned." I replied. "It's just a bad sunburn though, I'll be good."

Brian tilted his head to look at me seriously, "Do you know what sun poisoning is?" he asked.

I turned my whole body to face him since the collar of my shirt scraped painfully against my neck if I moved only my head, "Sun poisoning?" I said ignorantly.

Brian winced, "Oh dude... dude... sun poisoning is worse than just a sunburn. Way worse. How long were you out there?"

I looked down sheepishly at the ground, "A few hours..."

"Yeah, that's probably sun poisoning," He said with a slow nod, "You need a couple days off work dude."

Our boss ended up giving me a ride back to Uncle William's so I wouldn't have to walk home. I went straight to the couch and fell asleep. When I woke up, Donny and Uncle William were on the back patio talking and I could hear their voices in heated conversation together. I got up and headed out back to investigate.

"Think about your future, Donny." Uncle William pleaded.

"Man, I don't think that's how I wanna spend my time, being in court, working so closely with the law. Running a hydro shop sounds like a lot of fun.

Plus, I like plants." Donny replied, his voice uneasy and defensive.

Uncle William put his hands together, interlocking his fingers, "But think of how much more security you would have in this industry versus in a startup business that's on the less-than-legal side of things. A hydro shop is one thing on the outside, and another thing on the inside. I know you know what I'm talking about." Uncle William reasoned.

I lit a cigarette as I stepped out the door and sat down across the table from Donny. "You should really put some thought into this decision bubba." I said carefully. "It's not a decision you have to make right this second, but it's a big one."

Donny fidgeted with an empty pack of cigarettes, "I have thought about it. Why does everyone always think I'm making the worst choices? Why can't anyone ever just support me in what I want to do?" he lamented.

"We're trying to get you to make the right choice." Uncle William insisted.

"Bubba..." I started and paused to put my thoughts together carefully, "I love you. And I will support you no matter what you want to do." Those were the hardest words to say in that moment, and I hoped he appreciated how I tried to support him even when he was going to work for the guy who sexually abused me as a teenager. That bothered me intensely, but I still believed that I did something to deserve the abuse, so I compartmentalized it however I could to move on.

Uncle William sat back in his chair and gave me a death stare. I tried to ignore it and keep my attention on Donny.

"Thanks, man." Donnie nodded somberly and looked at me with a smile. "That's what I want to do. I want to go run the hydro shop." He assured me.

"What-the-hell-ever." Uncle William shook his head, fingers still interlocked.

Donny stood up, "Well, I gotta go get ready to help Tom again today. He should be here soon."

Uncle William nodded silently; his eyes locked on me.

I caught his gaze and addressed it, "What?" I said dryly.

"Thanks for fucking that up." His face was red. "When your brother ruins his life, that's on you and I hope you feel proud of yourself for it. Jesus fucking Christ..." He got up and stormed off.

I inhaled deeply and thought for a moment. What did Uncle William expect me to do? Donny was obviously decided on what he wanted to do, and we were just making him uncomfortable by berating him for it. I knew it was a better choice for him to work with Uncle William, but I also didn't want to make an enemy of my brother. Even if my brother had a rough path ahead, I wanted to be welcome in his life. At least I could be there and help when he needed it as long as I didn't draw some line in the sand over this. I was okay with that, at least. If I knew anything about people, it's that they were going to do exactly whatever they wanted regardless of how I felt or what I said about it and my brother was no exception to this rule.

The following weeks were a blur. Donny had taken his flight back to Memphis to work at the hydro shop, so I was stuck with Uncle William. The tension between us was out in the open and at an all-time high. He knew I was tired of his shit, and I knew he was tired of me. We avoided each other as much as possible, until the day it fell apart.

I walked through the back gate of Uncle William's driveway to have a seat at the glass table out back and have a cigarette after my 2-hour commute back from work. The sun had begun to set, so I appreciated the beautiful hues of bright pink and orange contrasted against the dark blue sky as I finished my cigarette.

Uncle William walked down the back patio steps from the house to come sit at the table with me. "Fuck... what now?" I whispered under my breath as I saw him approach.

Uncle William sat down and didn't say a word though. I planned to let that continue as long as it could, but the glorious silence was short-lived.

"This isn't working." He said and slid a plane ticket across the table to me. "You've gotta go back home. You're scheduled to leave next weekend and I'll drive you up to the airport."

A cacophony of emotions echoed and interacted in my mind, all competing for center stage. "Just... just like that?" The emotions spread across my facial features, and I couldn't help it.

"You've got to see that this isn't working." He lectured.

I shot forward in my seat, leaning over the table at him, "I'm days away from getting my first paycheck with the new raise. You know I went up almost

$4 an hour? That's enough for me to afford a cheap place here. We've got a buyer lined up for the house in Mississippi and they should be closing on that in a couple weeks. That's all I need, is a little more time. Can't you see that I'm working as quickly and hard as I can to get out of your hair? Do you think this is fun for me? I value my independence, and I've not had that in 3 months because of you. You've been going behind me and checking up on everything I do to make sure it's up to your approval and giving me copious amounts of shit for it if you don't like it." My frustration was welling up, but I made no effort to contain it.

I continued, "Not only that but you yell at me for spending my money, you yell at me for not spending my money, your decision forced me to walk 8 miles a day to work and 8 miles back. I have had to fight you this whole time, and now, when I'm so close to achieving my goal, you want to blow the whole thing up on me and remove my choice from the matter entirely. What the fuck, dude?"

Uncle William inhaled, "Oh don't put this on me." Nothing came across as clearly as his irritation in that moment.

I cocked my head sideways in confusion, "You mean, you don't want me..." I pointed to myself, "...to put your choices..." I pointed to him, "...on you?" I waggled my finger at him. "You're the one telling me I have no choice but to bow to your power move right now. How is this not on you? You bought me a plane ticket without saying a word to me about it. That's on you, no matter how much you want me to pretend otherwise."

He shrugged and stood up, "Yeah well you can live on the street if you want to stay in California, but you can't stay here anymore."

I put my first cigarette out and immediately pulled another from the pack, "So that's it then? You're kicking me out like this? What should I tell the people that want to buy my house?" I said loudly enough so he could hear me across the yard.

He just kept walking and didn't reply. I turned my attention back up toward the sunset. At least he couldn't take the sunset from me.

I looked down from the next sunset, which was just as beautiful as it was last night when I got my plane ticket. "Yeah," I said with a shrug, "He just ignored me and walked away." I grabbed a handful of beach sand, let gravity pull it back to the ground through my fingers, and shook my head in disappointment.

Brian patted me on the back, "Man, I'm really sorry. Is there anything we can do?"

I shook my head, "No, I don't think so. I can't afford to pay bills back home and also rent here. Not only that, but you guys have already done a lot for me. I don't think there's a way to make this work." I sighed, "Besides, I really miss my wife and just want to get back and see her. This has been such a long few months."

Nate stood up from the sand, winking at me with his bloodshot eye. "Let's get this bonfire going. The sun's almost down."

I stared into the bonfire for what felt like hours, trying to find my peace with the death of this California dream. The burning of the wood seemed almost symbolic. Smoke and ash.

Chapter 4

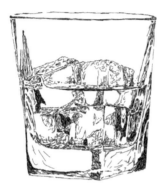

"Just then a tiny little dot caught my eye, it was just about too small to see, but I watched it way too long, and it was pulling me down..." Nine Inch Nails played again on my headphones, but the feeling of being above anything was absent this time.

I stared out of my window on the plane soberly. This plane ride sucked compared to the last one. What was everyone back home going to say? What would I tell them? What exactly happened anyway? What was so bad about me that I had to go with no explanation?

I had lots of questions and no answers to any of them. The answers had to be somewhere inside. Surely, with enough introspection, I'll be able to figure out where I went wrong and fix whatever it was that was so bad about me.

Once we had landed, Nashville felt surreal. I had been there before and had a wonderful time. This time though, the colors seemed a bit... duller almost. At least I was looking forward to seeing Liz again.

"Hey!" I heard Liz's voice up ahead in the baggage claim area, so I broke into a power walk in that direction. We met with a hug, and in that moment, I was whole again and could breathe. I could put the part of my brain to rest that had to figure out why I was defective, at least for now.

"I missed you so much." I put my forehead against hers, closed my eyes, and ran my fingers through her hair.

"I missed you, too. I'm so glad you're back." She whispered.

I took my bags out to the car and loaded them up, "You mind if I drive, babe?" I asked, knowing she didn't.

"Of course, it's all yours!" She tossed me the keys and got in the passenger's seat.

The ride home was quieter than I imagined it would be. Normally, I'd be talking non-stop about what's bothering me. I didn't understand the nuances that made the California move fall apart, but I felt like I could figure it out if I just kept picking at it.

Liz placed her hand on top of mine, "You okay? You're pretty quiet." She said thoughtfully. I could hear the genuine care in her voice that always made me feel like I was home.

I moved my thumb to stroke one of her fingers that draped down over my hand, "I'll be fine. I just... I'm trying to figure this out. This is the first time that I haven't been able to overcome the challenges in front of me. Normally I can just put more effort into something and it turns out fine. There has to be something I could have done differently, and I have to figure it out before I try something else. I still want a job in the tech sector." I shook my head, "If I can't figure out where I went wrong this time, how can I prevent it from happening again?"

Liz squeezed my hand, "It's ok, hun. I'm here if you need to talk about it." I could tell she was looking at me from my peripheral, but I kept my eyes on the road.

I inhaled deeply, trying to exhale the fog inside. "I... I don't even know where or how to start. I'm angry, I'm confused, I'm embarrassed, and... honestly, most of all, I'm..." I couldn't spit the word out, "I'm... I'm really insecure about it all." I started to tear up, but managed to control things enough so the dam didn't burst. I just breathed for a moment in silence. "I expected to finally leave this swampy hell behind." I looked at the forest of trees on either side of the Natchez Trace Parkway we were driving along. "I just... wanted out. I was so close to getting out, and Uncle William just pulled the rug out from under me. I thought he gave a shit and wanted to help. How could I have misunderstood him so badly. And how could I have been so misunderstood?" I wondered aloud.

Liz cocked her head with curiosity, "How were you misunderstood?" She asked sincerely.

I inhaled again, "Donny thought I was there to 'just hang out'. He told me so himself and I had to tell him why I was really there. And I still think he didn't really believe me after I told him." I shook my head in confusion. "And... I dunno... did Uncle William think the same thing somehow? And then, Uncle William yelled at me one day. He ran his short little ass right up to about an inch from my chest, all red-faced, and started yelling about not wiping the toilet seat."

"Oh..." Liz interjected with surprise.

I nodded, "Yeah, but the funny thing is, I wiped the toilet seat the last time I used the bathroom. I looked behind him at Donny and Donny was on the couch just watching Uncle William yell at me and I'm pretty sure he was the one who didn't wipe the seat. He just watched with this dumb look on his face."

"Did you tell Uncle William it wasn't you?" She asked sincerely.

I shook my head, eyes fixed on the road, "Nope, I took that one on the chin for Donny. And I'm pretty sure he doesn't even care."

Liz squeezed my hand again, "I'm sure he noticed."

I shrugged, "He may have noticed, but he didn't thank me or anything for it. He never talked about it again. It probably never even registered as a blip on his radar. Plus, I think he's making a mistake with this hydro shop with Samuel. Why did I even make contact with Samuel again? Jesus, I'm such an idiot." I lamented pathetically.

Liz's tone was instantly defensive, "You, Mr. Kester, are many things but an idiot is not one of them. That's an excuse you can't use with me because I know better." I could hear a smile come through her words at the end.

I needed to hear that, but I didn't want to hear it. I wanted to believe that I was idiot, but that was just depression creeping in. "You're not wrong..." I replied, "But... damn it, this whole thing just sucks and I don't know where to put all the pieces... I know it all fit together at one point, but how did this happen? Going back to work is going to be embarrassing. We had to tell the people who wanted to buy our house, 'Never mind,'" I feigned my best caveman voice, "'Just kidding, no sell house.' You know? Uncle William doesn't really give a shit about any of that. He just wanted me gone. Like..." I inhaled, "What the fuck was so terrible that I had to go?" We finished the trip and arrived home, but that question continued to haunt me.

I repeated that same question to Uncle William, weeks later, over the phone. "Look man, it's eating me up. What was so bad about me that I had to go immediately?" I asked him calmly, feeling confident that we could get somewhere discussing this like adults.

A moment of silence passed before he yelled, "You know, I don't know why you haven't gotten the hell over this yet! Move on, for fuck's sake!"

I was surprised. I thought we had a decent conversation talking about the past few weeks of work. I'd obviously hit a button to change his cadence entirely like this. I let the silence hang in the air as I tried not to respond in anger. "Fuck you..." the words echoed in my head, but I couldn't let them fall out of my mouth. "Okay. Alright." I said as calmly as I could. "I'm over it. Talk to ya later." And I hung up the phone. I decided I would never talk to that man again in my life if I can help it. I don't want to see him, hear him, or think about him. I murdered his memory that night, sitting on my front porch.

It only seemed fitting to mourn the loss of a childhood hero, so I grabbed a glass of whiskey, headed to my front porch, and tried to remember the good moments.

"Oh no," Uncle William protested, waggling one finger and looking at Mom over the top of his sunglasses, "We're not buying this 6-year-old boy a gun, even if it is a toy."

I looked at the nerf gun on the store shelf, then again at Uncle William. I'd felt sorry for asking mom if I could have it.

"Oh, it's a nerf gun, William... I don't see what th-" Mom was almost laughing, so surely, she wasn't really in trouble.

"No, it's still a gun. You point it at people, you pull a trigger, it shoots a projectile at them. When you get back to Colorado, you can buy him whatever you want. But while you're out here... no guns." He had a little sass to him, but dropped the sass and turned to me, "I'm sorry, Lenny. You

see, I don't like guns. In fact, I believe very passionately that the whole world would be a better place if nobody had any guns at all, even toy guns. I think that instead of teaching our children to compete against each other with toy guns, it would be better if we taught them how to work together to create new things that wouldn't exist otherwise." He looked around the aisle we were on for a second, then looked back at me, "Here. I'll show you what I mean."

Uncle William walked back to the end of the aisle and looked up and down the rows at the signs. "Come on, come check this out." Uncle William waved Mom and I over to him.

"Here, what about this?" Uncle William held out an evil scientist play kit. It had a picture of Frankenstein on it, had a couple of beakers and flasks, and you used the equipment to make rubber creatures out of molds like snakes, spiders, scorpions, and centipedes.

My eyes lit up as I grabbed the box from Uncle William and began looking at all the pictures on the back of the box, "Ohhhh! This is soooo cooooool Mom!!" Little me exclaimed., practically bouncing up and down.

Uncle William looked up at Mom with a smile, "My treat."

I smiled and sipped my whiskey. I still prefer cooperative activities over competitive activities to this day. I wonder if that has anything to do with my current disposition. I searched for another good memory.

The San Diego streets were filled with people watching the parade go by. Laughter, cheering, and encouragement filled the air. "Oh my god..." I laughed, "This is wild... dykes on bikes? Like, look, they have a sign that says, 'Dykes on Bikes' on all their motorcycles!" I pointed and clapped. "That's magnificent!" Most of the women had biceps and triceps alone that put my whole body to shame. I was 16, so I had acne. I was tall and lanky. I was skinny and pale. Those self-proclaimed dykes on bikes would have snapped me like a twig. It was truly impressive.

Then came the 'Boy Toys' section of the parade. Topless guys in colorful skirts twirled batons with streamers. Some even did somersaults.

People from all walks of life around the city showed support for the *queer folk. It was like stepping into another reality where people accepted each other for their weird differences. It felt really good to know that all these people were being exactly who they wanted to be without social consequences. That was an experience that just didn't exist in Memphis.*

I sipped my whiskey again and smiled. That Gay Pride Parade was instrumental in shaping my attitude and I was glad for it. I was sure I was a better, more well-rounded person for having the experience. And I had Uncle William to thank for that. "To the dead," I said under my breath and raised my glass before taking another sip of whiskey. Another memory was coming into focus.

"So, I just laid there and pretended to be asleep because I didn't know what to do. I was like... frozen or something." I was telling Uncle William about my first sexual encounter because I didn't know who else to turn to.

Uncle William sat down on the couch next to me, "Well, did you have an orgasm?" He asked plainly.

"Well... yes, but... I don't know, I didn't want that to happen. I'm just now exploring my sexuality, and even that's hard because mom's so religious." I shook my head, "And like, I don't know if I'm gay... I like girls still... Sure, some guys are really good-looking, but men are so... aggressive." I mused.

"Have you talked to him about it yet?" Uncle William asked.

I shook my head, "No, we don't really ever talk about it and what it's become."

Uncle William looked concerned, "It's become something? What's it become?"

I shrugged and winced, "I dunno, I just haven't mentioned it and it's happened a few more times. And like, I'm not really okay with it, but I don't want to nuke the whole friendship... I want the friendship we had before the sexual stuff started..."

Uncle William grabbed one of his cats that had just jumped up on the couch next to him, "It sounds like you care about him. How does being in a homosexual relationship make you feel?" He asked calmly.

I paused for thought for a moment before answering, "I do care about him. I care about lots of people though and it never becomes sexual. The idea of being in a gay relationship honestly doesn't bother me if I found the right person. Maybe I'm just picky and I don't belong with Samuel, but men seem too greedy and disconnected to make any kind of meaningful connection with. But what do I do with these feelings inside about all the sexual stuff? I don't know how to be okay with what's going on with Samuel and I."

Uncle William looked at me calmly and said, "You have to talk to him about it."

"But he's not an open, reasonable person most of the time. He carries around a lot of hurt, and I want to be there for him and not run away like everyone else did, but he just argues with me so much about everything." I started sobbing.

Uncle William put his hand on my shoulder, "Look, there's nothing wrong with being gay. But if you're not comfortable in that relationship, you need to address it with him and make a change in your life or it won't ever go away on its own."

I looked out from my front porch and sipped my whiskey again. Uncle William was right all those years ago, and I eventually did make a change that separated me from Samuel. I had Uncle William to thank for that too. There was a lot of hurt and confusion because I honestly never really talked about it with Samuel back then. I never felt like I could trust Samuel with the truth because he would always argue with me when I gave it to him. It got bad before I finally pulled the plug and ended the relationship all those years ago.

A sliver of light grew from the front door as Liz opened it and found me. "Hey, there you are. Whatcha doin' out here?" Liz's soft voice broke the silence.

"Just burying an old hero," I replied somberly and took another sip of whiskey.

She stepped out onto the front porch, "What happened?"

I told her about the conversation with Uncle William from earlier in the evening. "So, this is me getting over it." I raised my empty glass of whiskey. "To an old hero."

I tried going with Liz when she went back to bed, but I couldn't sleep. I couldn't get the situation figured out. Did I overreact to Uncle William? It felt like he only wanted to hear certain things when we talked on the phone – pleasantries only, please, but nothing real. He snapped when I asked him about what happened, so I was clearly never going to get a straightforward answer. Everything was so fresh on my mind, I had to write some sort of poem to let it all out. I got back up and wrote whatever I felt like writing.

You ask how I'm doing?
I'll tell you: it's ruing.

The waters of hope and trust,
Stagnant, stale, and full of disgust,
Sulfur, poison, cancer, and rust,
Saturating my mouth and lungs like dust.

Intoxicating hubris and cunning speech,
Ruminating on pretentious words that taste like bleach,
Inured to pernicious ideology,
Gaining heavy momentum into despondency.

Whatever happened to peace and love?
Concepts that faded in the push and shove,
Lost in the disorientation thereof,
I'm losing distance between here and above.

Pining, withered, faded, and forgotten,
Lacking the strength to reverse the rotten,
Overwhelming chagrin subverting my dreams,
My livelihood is dissolving at the seams.

But sympathy is obnoxious, so I'll keep on masking,
The pain I can't move past, my heart notwithstanding,
In every possible way, I'm lacking,
But sure, I'm doing well, thanks for asking.

I woke up the next morning to my phone ringing. I saw it was Liz and answered it, "Hey babe. What's up?"

"Heyyyyyy" She started sweetly, "I'm gonna ask you a thing. You can totally say no if you really want to, but... but... honey... there's a baby puppy up here that needs a home and he is so cute and fluffy and precious and sweet and we can't just let him go in the parking lot or he's going to get ran over, and I would feel-" She was excited, and I could tell because she was talking very fast.

I stopped her, "Babe... babe... yes, of course it's ok. If that puppy needs a home, we can give it one."

"OH THANK YOU!! YAY!" Excitement and laughter burst through my phone. "Ohh, this makes me SO happy. Ok... ok... AHHHHHH I GET TO KEEP THE PUPPY!!" She sounded like she was shouting to someone else in the background, "Ok sorry, um... Sloan has the precious baby puppy now. She just found him in the parking lot but can't keep him. We got him a box, and Sloan took him to her house to get him some food and a blanket. I'll bring him home with me tonight."

And like that, we had our first dog. Potty training him and being depressed was an interesting combination, but we made it through. We named him Mobius and called him Moby for short. When he wasn't peeing on the floors, he was my best lil buddy.

The following months were filled with plenty of poor decisions that stemmed from the worsening depression. Depression had been tightening its grip since coming back to Mississippi, and I knew it. I quit the Geek Squad for 100 different reasons, but it came down to quitting before I got fired. The new manager and I bumped heads a lot and had a few heated conversations. Those conversations landed me my first write-ups at the company, and it was a matter of time before my worsening attitude made that situation uninhabitable for me.

I found some success independently helping medical clinics get their old paper records transferred over to electronic records and fixing their small issues along the way. Over time, I had become the IT guy for a couple of clinics by doing this.

I walked past one of my client's offices and noticed that she was scrolling through Dodge's website, building a brand new Charger. I went back to supervise her new high-speed internet connection. She had just upgraded from dial-up internet, which I didn't know anyone still provided service for in 2013, to cable internet services and I needed to oversee the whole process. She was upgrading per the new HIPPA guidelines, and I was setting her up with the new process for transferring all her old paper records into electronic records.

I was getting frustrated with her though, because she would argue with me when I told her what she needed, and then when I would try and make concessions to see if I could get her older technology working with the newer technology, it wouldn't work, and I would have to tell her that we have no choice but to spend more money. She would get aggravated any time she had to invest in her computer systems. She was still using Windows 95 on the majority of computers in her office, so I knew she didn't like to change things very often. If being HIPPA compliant didn't require a reliable high-speed internet connection, she wouldn't have upgraded from dial-up.

I finished supervising the internet installation and came back to her office, where she was still browsing the Dodge website. I knocked on her door and looked at the ground. She minimized the website and turned around in her office chair to face me, "Yeah, what's up?" She asked in an old, raspy voice.

I approached her desk, "The guys from the cable company can't get your server computer to connect. It comes down to an IP conflict, but you're going to have this issue every time you restart that server machine unless we upgrade you to a newer operating system." I explained.

She put some reading glasses on, "So what's that mean then? I gotta spend more money?"

I'd had this conversation with her a few times already, so I knew she was about to get shitty and start arguing with me. "Well, the choice is yours. You can call me out here every time you restart your server machine, or you can buy a new server that won't have that issue."

"I paid you to get me HIPPA compliant, and I'm not HIPPA compliant yet! You keep coming back to me telling me I need to spend more money and not getting me HIPPA compliant!" She argued like a spoiled schoolkid.

"Ma'am, I understand what we're trying to do. I hope you understand that your computer systems are seriously outdated, and you have a lot of updating to do in order to fully meet HIPPA compliance. I'm trying my hardest to make what you have work, but I'm running into lots of unexpected limitations and I'm probably going to continue running into lots more."

I desperately needed her to understand that I could not make windows 95 machines do all the same things that newer Windows 7 machines could do without lots of crazy workarounds that were going to cost me more time than I wanted to spend and cost her more money than she wanted to spend, but she didn't want to hear it.

"Ma'am, the government is giving you $120,000 through the new HIPPA program exactly for this reason. Upgrading computer systems is costly an-" Uh oh...

She sprang up out of her chair and stood in front of me, "You don't come in here and tell me how to spend MY money!" She yelled at the top of her lungs. "I paid you $500 to get me HIPPA compliant and you keep trying to get all my money!" She stomped righteously.

I looked at her, then I looked at her computer monitor where she had minimized the Dodge website, and I suddenly understood what I had stepped in. I looked back at her, "I'll tell you what, ma'am, you find someone else who is willing to upgrade your Windows 95 systems to modern technology for $500 and get them to come get you HIPPA compliant, because I'm not your guy." And I turned and walked out.

I decided that running my own computer repair business was riskier than I was okay with. Nowhere did I sign any contracts with that lady, nor did I have any legal protection if something went wrong with her old computer systems. As old as her computers were, it was only a matter of time before something went wrong.

I had nothing after that. No plan, no money saved up, just a sign in the front yard that said, "computer repair" and had my cell phone number on it. I got no calls, and I eventually took the sign down. Unchecked, because I refused to acknowledge it, my depression had grown, day by day, stronger and stronger, for nearly a year since I had gotten home from California.

I approached my wife at my lowest point one day. "I think we should separate," I said, knowing there was really no good way to broach this topic.

Liz looked at me with concern and started to respond but started crying.

God, I was so confused... I wasn't trying to hurt her, but I needed to find myself. I was so lost in the storm of my own depression, that I felt like I couldn't be the husband she needed, but I had no clue how to communicate that. I felt so guilty for being so overcome with my own emotions. I had no direction. No motivation to do anything else, professionally speaking. I felt like a cancer, and I was trying to not let it spread to Liz, or that's what I told myself anyway. I needed some time to figure things out. I'd figure it out along the way...

"I still love you, and I don't necessarily want a divorce, and I don't want you completely out of my life, but I just need some space right now. I'm lost and I can't be what you need me to be." I started crying. "I need to find myself before I do something stupid out of depression." I feared suicide, to be honest. It scared the hell out of me.

Sobbing, Liz replied, "If that's what you feel like you need to do, I won't stop you." She was definitely upset and for good reason. I felt even worse now, but at least a little bit hopeful that I could find myself again. I really had no plan; I was just reacting very poorly to my emotions...

Chapter 5

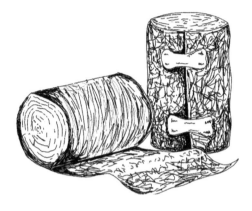

I woke up and stretched in bed. I was alone, and I missed both Liz and Moby, but I had to 'find myself,' whatever the hell that meant. I rolled over to look at my phone for the date. The days blended together when you didn't have a job. It didn't really matter whether it was Tuesday, Wednesday, or Friday – every day was the same. But it was a Friday, after all, whatever that matters for.

I got up and showered. My hair was long now, and it always amazed me how much extra shampoo was needed. Long hair is expensive, and I get it now. I put my hair into a ponytail, put one of my pairs of Thai fishermen's pants on, grabbed a t-shirt, slipped on my flip-flops, and headed out to the kitchen to make some coffee.

"Good morning, dude!" JP said to me as he rushed back to his bedroom. JP was a little younger than me, but had already started to lose some hair, so he just shaved his head bald. He had a long, full beard that reached down to his chest.

I smiled, "Good morning, man!" I hollered back down the hallway and continued my caffeine conquest for the morning.

After making coffee, I went into my room and logged on to ESO (Elder Scrolls Online), this new MMO that was in BETA testing and would be released in a few weeks. I was a long-time Elder Scrolls fan, so of course I had to be there from the beginning for this one. I logged on to my main character and continued exploring and leveling, finding bugs, and submitting feedback about the leveling experience. It was a good distraction during that time.

I got up and came out for coffee when I heard it beep.

"Morning!" Ingram said as he rushed into the kitchen for some coffee. Ingram was also bald. He shaved as well, and together he and JP were the Bald and Beautiful crew. Ingram was clean-shaven and had no facial hair.

"Good morning, man!" I cheerily replied. I walked up to the coffee pot and JP joined us. "Here we gather today, oh almighty caffeine, in need of your strength to start another day..." I held my hands up like I was in church and bowed my head.

JP and Ingram both busted out in laughter. Ingram continued, "We are humbled by your awesome powers, and promise not to take them in vain. Now get in my veins!" He laughed.

"Seriously, I don't know what I'd do without caffeine..." JP thought respectfully.

"Yeah, me either... All hail caffeine!" I kept it going.

"All hail caffeine!" We said in unison, and off to work they went. We were goofy, but we didn't care. It was fun. JP had been my best friend since I was 14, and he'd met the man of his dreams in Ingram. Anyone that made JP that happy was ok in my book.

After they had gone to work for the day, I sat down at my computer and drank some coffee in my room, played some ESO, and spent plenty of time waking up. Once I had gotten some caffeine in my system, I put my headphones in, picked a room, and cleaned it. Today's room was the living room. Not that JP and Ingram's place was a mess, but if I didn't keep the place clean, they would have to spend their time doing it. I wanted to make sure their time off was free from stuff like that since I had all the time in the world. Plus, I like us being able to dedicate the weekend to gaming and not to cleaning. I could clean up throughout the week, and that, by itself, was good for me if only for discipline's sake. There was no reason not to clean up throughout the week, in my mind.

I dusted first, which alerted the cats to what always followed – the vacuum.

I put a few dirty cups in the sink and cleaned off all the tables and the cats started to slink out of the living room quietly. They anxiously watched me from as far away as possible as I dusted from top to bottom and cleaned all the surfaces. They would get bored and wander up to me and the cleaning supplies, and I would totally stop cleaning for a minute to pet the cats.

But then came the vacuum. The cats now considered me enemy number one, but I wasn't done until the carpet had those nice uniform vacuum marks in it. After vacuuming, I set some incense out and put a lighter next to it. I'd light that later, right before JP and Ingram get home. And of course, the cats are laying across the freshly vacuumed carpet, depositing fresh fur.

Time for the kitchen. The kitchen was a daily thing unless we ate out the night before. I started with the dishes. That was always the part I disliked the most in the kitchen, so might as well get it out of the way first, then it's downhill from there. I wiped the counters down with disinfectant, refreshed the pets' water bowls and cleaned their area up. By then, the dishes were dry, so I put them away before going over the floor with a wet Swiffer.

Then I logged back on to ESO, hopped into Discord voice chat, and queued up for PvP.

"Yo! Sup guys?" I asked my clanmates over the Discord voice chat.

"Alessia is under siege and it's the last emperor keep. We gotta dethrone this piece of trash today!" Koni said.

"X-up in chat, Icky, I'll pick you up in the main group. We need all the bodies we can get to take this keep. We're going to have to punch multiple breaches in the outer wall to get in, and most likely breach both inner postern doors." Agrippa announced calmly. If anyone ever had a voice that embodied "ideal leadership" in both tone and style, it was Agrippa's voice. He enunciated clearly, spoke quickly, and meant exactly what he said.

"Bet." I answered. I made sure I had plenty of buff food on my character, plenty of healing and utility potions, and plenty of siege equipment, and checked that all my gear was in order. Preparation was important because I couldn't run out of basic consumables during the middle of a fight. That would make me a weak link in the team.

I met up with my group in the golden fields of Cyrodiil, and we sieged that keep in a 100 vs. 100 vs. 100, 3-way battle for nearly 4 hours before achieving victory. Some of the fights were long, but it was those big fights that we chased. There was never a moment where 10-30 of us weren't together in combat, trying to manage our distances from each other, trying out different group tactics, communicating and coordinating attacks on other players, and regrouping to heal the wounded.

We would have discussions about different group compositions and builds and the different things we could achieve in certain situations by min/maxing our resources as a group. The possibilities seemed endless, and we kept coming up with new ways to outmaneuver or outmatch our enemies.

Once JP and Ingram got home from work for the day, I logged out and joined them in the living room to discuss dinner.

JP put both hands on his cheeks and pulled down, stretching his face out a little, "Hmmm... I dunno, anything sounds good right now. I'm just hungry. I'd eat anything you put in front of me. I'm not picky." JP said, casting his vote for dinner.

Ingram rolled his eyes and laughed, "What about Zaxby's Chicken?" He asked.

"That does sound good..." I commented. "I'm also hungry and would eat whatever was put in front of me, but Zaxby's does sound good."

"I'm perfectly happy with Zaxby's, babe." JP bowed his head politely at Ingram.

"All right, let's pack up and go get it." Ingram grabbed the keys and tossed them to JP.

We all packed into JP's Black 2009 Honda Civic SI Coupe. The windows were tinted, it had an aftermarket spoiler, a body kit, and red trim around body. As far as Civics go, this thing looked mean. It was a manual transmission, so JP would drive it like he stole it. And, honestly, in Memphis, that's par for the course.

The time we spent in the line was longer than the time it took to drive there and back, but we had our hot, delicious chicken and could go home and nest in for the night.

"Oh man, you guys should come play some ESO with me soon! It's a lot of fun." I set my empty Zaxby's container on the coffee table and sat back on the couch.

JP took a bite of his chicken, "Mmm, yeah, you know I was gonna download it and check it out. I might do that soon."

Ingram nodded, wiping his mouth with a napkin, "It does look kinda cool. It could be fun. I'll probably try it eventually." He took another bite and then suddenly looked like he remembered something. After hurriedly chewing, he wiped his mouth again and said, "So guess what I found today..."

JP and I both fixed our attention on him, "What?" we said, nearly in unison.

"An anvil. An -ANVIL-," He burst out in laughter, "Someone left it in their apartment after they moved out. Who just has this stuff lying around their apartment?" He mused.

"Hahaha," JP laughed, "An anvil? Like a medieval blacksmith's anvil?" JP stared at Ingram in disbelief.

Ingram nodded slowly, "A whole-ass anvil!"

"What did you guys do with it?" I asked, overcome with curiosity.

"Well..." Ingram started, "The first thing I did was ask my manager if I could keep it..." his voice trailed off.

"...and?" JP asked expectantly.

"..Aaaand now I have to figure what to do with an anvil." Ingram couldn't contain the burst of laughter that followed.

"Oh my god..." JP put his hand on his cheek, "You didn't..."

Ingram nodded, face red with laughter.

"You find some crazy shit around this place, don't you Ingram?" I asked through my own laughter.

"Damn right I do. Like, these people are into all kinds of shit." He shook his head and paused for a second before remembering something, "Oh yeah, don't forget this weekend is the pool party. I've got to be there since I'm on the staff, but we're hosting it for the residents. You should at least come down and get some free beer and a free burger. Everyone loves free beer and free food, right?"

Yeah, he was right. Everyone loves free beer and food, and I was no exception. I went there for free stuff, but so did everyone else. As the pool party went on, I noticed that everyone seemed to be treating it like a competition to see who could drink the most before the apartment complex ran out of beer.

I wasn't participating in the unspoken contest, but I also wasn't showing any reserve in my drinking. We'd been there a couple of hours, and I was being boring. I was staying at our table, drinking beer, and hadn't gotten up once. I really had no interest in making friends or socializing, I was just there because JP and Ingram were there and there was free beer.

The apartment manager was wearing a generic black apron and cooking hamburgers and hotdogs on the grill over on the far side of the pool. Just then, I noticed one of the female tenants standing by the grill looking at me. She was wearing a tank top and some shorts. As she got closer, I could see that she was pretty.

Oh no... she was actually approaching me and probably noticed me looking at her. I had no clue what I was going to say or do. I felt pressure to respond amicably, but I was nervous. I had wanted the opportunity to date someone else to see how different it was from Liz. This could be my chance, but did I really want anyone but Liz? Also, dating sucked and I'd forgotten how bad it sucked until that moment when I was trying to figure out how I felt and what to say.

She approached my table and waved, "This seat taken?" She pointed to a seat right across the table from me.

I shook my head, "No, it's all yours." I smiled pleasantly and took a gulp of beer.

JP looked at me with a smirk before answering her, "No. Please, have a seat." He tipped his beer toward the empty seat.

We talked for over an hour about the weather, our food preferences, exercise habits, hobbies, and professional interests. And the whole time, underneath the entire conversation, was a vague blanket of apprehension. I didn't understand why I was feeling this way. Wasn't this what I wanted? She was pretty, but the longer we talked, the stronger that feeling grew.

"So... hey..." She started softly, almost seductively. "I gotta walk to Kroger around the corner, you wanna come with?"

I thought for a moment. We had been pounding beers for the last hour and we were both fairly drunk. And she was a pretty lady. It wasn't painting a good situation, walking around the streets of Memphis alone like that. By this point though, I knew I didn't want this to turn into anything. I wanted to get back to my computer and play some ESO. But then I also felt guilty for telling this drunk woman to go to Kroger on her own.

I chugged the last third of my beer and threw the bottle into a nearby trash can, "Yeah," I swallowed, "I'll walk with you. I could stand to walk off some of this alcohol." I wondered if there was a way to communicate that I was just being nice and wasn't hoping for a score. Talking to someone was one thing, but I wasn't wanting to sleep around.

I let JP know that I would be back in a few minutes. We got up from the table and I followed her away from the pool area.

She turned her head sideways toward me, not changing her forward pace, "I have to stop by my apartment first and get my wallet." She stumbled slightly.

I winced upon noticing the stumble, "Yeah, ok." I answered calmly, but I was panicking inside. She was drawing me into her lair.

We got to her place, and she walked toward the back, I assumed toward her room, "You can come... back... if you want, I'm just gonna... change my shoes and... find my wallet." Her words were slow, and she labored through the alcohol to push them out with clarity. The struggle was obvious.

I waited in the front room for a few minutes, but I noticed I stopped hearing noises from back there in her room. Concerned, I called back there, "Hey, how's it going?"

No reply. I wondered if maybe she took something and OD'd back there. My mind went crazy with different worst-case scenarios, each idea trying to top the previous idea in terribleness. "Hey," I called out a little louder this time, "You good back there?"

I heard a very faint, "Mm-hmm..." followed by some mumbles. I couldn't tell what she was saying from where I was in the front room. I inhaled deeply, somehow feeling drawn to take each next step leading someplace I knew I didn't want to be, literally and figuratively.

I walked down the hall toward the room she went into. The door was open, so I put my head down and looked at the ground before stepping up to the doorway and knocking on the frame.

"Heyyy..." she moaned, "Come over, Kroger can wait." Her voice sounded like she was high almost.

I looked up and saw her laying on her back on her bed, wearing nothing but a pair of pink lingerie panties. She waved her matching pink bra gently with one outstretched hand, like the white flag of surrender.

I saw no way out of this except to just say what needed to be said. I inhaled, "Hey, I'm sorry... you're very pretty, and in another situation, I would love to do this right now. But, I can't. I just can't. Not only am I deciding whether to get back with my wife or not, but you're very drunk and I don't want to feel like I took advantage of that. I'm just gonna head back home and hope our paths cross again soon." I smiled, feeling like I'd done a good job of addressing the situation.

"Aww, come onnn..." she protested sexily, "I'm right here." She held both arms out.

Holy crap... she's not giving up. She must be -REALLY- drunk. I wondered if she would remember any of this in the morning, "Hey, look, I want you to know that it's taking every bit of willpower not to have a lot of fun with you right now. You're gorgeous and sexy, but I'm just not in a place for that right now. I am truly... very sorry." I tried my best to look her in her eyes sincerely. The craziest challenge of my life in that moment...

She dropped her arms, blinked semi-consciously a few times, and I think immediately passed out. I turned to walk out, "See you around I hope!" I said quickly, locking the doorknob and shutting her front door behind me.

I inhaled deeply and exhaled slowly outside her front door before getting my bearings and heading back to JP and Ingram's place.

I was on the other side of the apartment complex, so I decided to jog. As I was running past the tennis court, my foot found a hole about 10 inches deep. I didn't see the hole coming because it had been mowed over, so all the thick grass there was the same height.

CRUNCH

I went down, tumbling forward with the momentum of my jog. Pain shot up from my foot before I had even hit the ground. I laid there for a second, just feeling the pain and trying to gain some mental clarity. I looked down at my ankle, and it was already red and swollen a little bit. I sat up and lifted my leg. As my ankle dangled, it moved ever so slightly and sent sharp spikes of pain up my leg.

"Oooooooooooooooooo..." I groaned and pulled my leg up to try and prop my foot into a comfortable position. After a few minutes of trying and finding no success making my ankle comfortable, I decided to try and walk home. I had to pass back by the pool, so maybe JP was still there and could help me back to the house.

Still drunk, I tried hopping on one foot back to the pool area. It wasn't far from where I was, so I just had to push through the pain and hobble there. I stopped a couple of times to lean against trees and rest, but eventually made it to the pool. JP was still sitting at the table, so I tried walking as normally as possible and sat down next to him.

I was focusing on my breathing and not getting sick from the pain. I must not have been able to keep the pain from expressing itself through my face, because JP immediately knew something was wrong.

"Woah, hey man are you ok? You look pale as a ghost. Did you go to Kroger?" JP said, full of surprise.

I moved my eyes only to look at JP, wincing "Man..." I breathed in pain, "...that was some kind of little adventure..." I breathed in pain again, "...and I think I fucked up my ankle pretty good."

JP scooted his chair back slightly and sat up, "Oh man, are you ok? Do we need to take you to the hospital? What happened?"

I put my weight on my good foot and hopped over to the chair to face JP, "Here, look. I stepped in a hole while I was coming back here just now." I breathed in pain as I grabbed my thigh with both hands and assisted the injured ankle into place in front of JP so he could see it.

JP leaned forward to inspect the ankle. "Jesus, dude, I'm not even going to pull the sock down. Your ankle is swollen up like a grapefruit. Hang on." He got up and ran off.

I rubbed my swollen ankle softly and grew more worried.

JP came back, "Okay, Len, Ingram's on the way over. He's gonna help you get home and into bed. Man, that looks bad..." He sat down in front of me again, "Ingram knows one of the other staff members who is EMT certified. He's going to see if they can come to look at it, too."

I winced, "Thanks man. Feels like I fucked it up pretty good."

"Hey! You ok man?" Ingram's voice grew closer from behind.

I turned my head to look back at him. As he came into my view, he started, "JP said you fucked your ank- Oh..." He was close enough that he could see it now. "Damn. Glad I have Amber coming to look at it. Let's get you home.

C'mon, can you grab onto my shoulder?"

Ingram helped me hobble back home and sat me in bed, "Hang on, I'll go find out where Amber is." He said and rushed back off. I sat up and swung my injured ankle onto the bed.

Ingram came back a few moments later with Amber. "Hey," Amber said with a thick southern accent, "Heard you took a nasty fall and hurt your ankle real good?"

I nodded in pain, "Yeah I was jogging in the grass and stepped into a hole..." I trailed off, rubbing my swollen ankle gently.

"Hopefully, you just sprained it real good. Lemme look at it." She held her hand out, so I swung my ankle around for her to inspect. She gently pressed into the swollen area and moved the ankle itself around in a very slow, controlled, and torturous manner. It hurt, but we ended up determining that it was most likely just a sprained ankle.

"Here, I brought some things that might be helpful." She opened a big orange and white pack of supplies and pulled a wrap and a cold pack out. She wrapped my ankle with the compressive cloth roll, put the cold gel pack around my ankle, wrapped a thick towel around that, and told me to lay down so that my ankle was resting on the cold pack. "If the swelling doesn't start going down in a day or two, or you notice any weird discoloration to the ankle area, go to the hospital immediately." She finished wrapping my ankle and handed out some final instructions.

I passed out right after she left and slept for the rest of the afternoon. There goes my sleep schedule...

Chapter 6

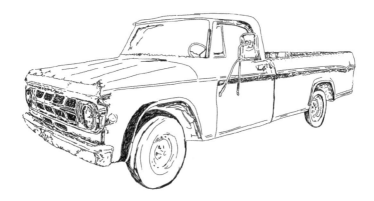

I quietly survey my prey from a safe distance and height inside the walled Imperial City of Cyrodiil. The target was a member of an opposing faction, and he was rifling through crates looking for goods to pilfer, no doubt. He walked around to destroyed horse carts, searching the debris for anything usable. I waited for my moment to attack and took it.

"It was just one." I reported. "I got him." I scouted ahead for the group often, providing info back to our leader.

Just then, I spotted a massive group of enemies headed our way. They had all started pouring out of a door not far up ahead. They would be here fast. I sprinted as quickly as I could back to my group, who was charging toward me into that same room.

"My batswarm ulti on crown now, large group incoming immediately. At least 20, maybe 30." I announced over Discord voice. I was running a dangerous distance ahead of the safety of my friends, but I always enjoyed playing it risky. High risk, high reward.

"My standard," Agrippa, or 'crown' as we referred to him since he led the group, knew I saw something big and began preparing. "All ults on me, all ults on crown now!" He ordered us as he saw the group of enemies rounding the corner in front of us.

Our groups collided violently, and they ran straight into all of our ultimate abilities. The entire enemy group immediately died.

"Hahahaha! Wow, that was perfect timing," Gomer sounded like he was bouncing up and down in his computer chair on the other side of Discord.

"Ha ha ha!" Agrippa laughed, "They were not as prepared as we were. That was a meatgrinder!"

"Wow, that was so perfect, I bet they're still trying to figure out what happened." I joked.

Just then I got a text from Ingram, "Samuel's out front, asked to talk to ya real quick. I gotta get back to work".

Shit... I never knew how to talk to Samuel. I hated him, but I had to be nice and keep things copasetic for my brothers' sake.

"Ok guys, I gotta log out for a bit but I'll be back on later." I announced over Discord.

"See ya, Icky." The soft roar of 14 voices echoed at me through Discord. It made me smile. I enjoyed all the time I put into Player vs Player combat with my group of online friends. We would plan for battles and come up with new strategies together when we weren't actively fighting. We would get into castle fights for hours, all of us listening to Agrippa's orders and murdering droves of our enemies.

Those successes, digital as they were, brought us together as friends. We had to learn to work together and overcome the challenges we faced as a team. We learned from our failures. We spent time preparing, planning, and synergizing with each other. Stuck in depression, my friends were a lifeline. We could come together and do our thing without all the weight of our personal lives. None of that mattered there if you could perform in combat. I was good at this, and it could distract me long enough to let the daily depression wear off so I could cook and clean and function.

But suddenly now, I had to go figure out what Samuel wanted. That was the thing about Samuel, he always wanted something out of you. If he didn't tell you, then he expected you to just know somehow and he would berate you until it really sank in.

I put my shoes on and walked out to the parking lot to meet Samuel. I could already feel my heartbeat picking up. Conversations with him always got intense and made me anxious.

Samuel rolled down the heavily tinted window of his truck and stuck his arm through the opening, revealing a lit cigarette, "Yo. Get in." He spoke with authority. He was wearing a black hoodie and dark sunglasses. The hood was down, revealing his short, dark brown hair. He was about 320 pounds and acted like a thug.

I inhaled. This won't be fun... What the hell did he want anyway? I'm pretty sure he thought I was useless, at least he told me so last time we spoke.

I walked around the truck and grabbed the handle of the door, questioning my sanity. I pulled the door handle up until I felt resistance and stopped. Why was I getting into the truck with him? I knew I didn't want to. I knew nothing good was going to come of it. Not many people scare me, but he legitimately does and always has. Like he could murder me and feel nothing about it if I said the wrong thing to him on the wrong day. Was today the wrong day?

I clicked the door handle up with an exhale and the door opened slowly. I climbed into the tall truck, "What's up?" I said, knowing the amount of energy I was putting into trying not to sound anxious was obvious.

"Yo, close the door, let's go." He commanded sternly.

I blinked then looked at him, "Where are we going?"

His head dipped forward and hung there, "For a ride, fucker." He snapped back. "Close the damn door! Fuckin' hate repeatin' myself. You know that."

Jesus Christ, I hated being talked to like that. On top of the anxiety, I was getting agitated. I could already see a bad trajectory forming here, just like it did so many times in the past. I decided to go with the flow and closed the door, against my better judgment. "So... what's up?" I asked nervously.

Samuel nodded, "So Alex been down here with Donny for a lil while now. It's not going good. Alex is addicted to pills and won't quit fuckin' around and I'm about to dump his ass back up to Indiana where he can live with his junkie friends in junkie paradise. I won't put up with this shit."

Oh boy... I put my head down, "He certainly keeps things interesting, doesn't he? Does he want to go back to Indiana? What does he want to do?"

Samuel put the truck in drive and pulled off. "I don't fuckin' care what he wants! He's not pullin' his weight." He was sounding quite agitated.

I inhaled slowly, trying to ease my anxiety and focus on this new development with Alex, "Sounds like he's maybe just not into that work. Like it's not motivating him? Maybe he does need to go back to Indiana. We should have a conversation with him about it." I replied thoughtfully.

Samuel shook his head, eyes fixed on the road, "Oh, hell naw. I tried talkin' to him. His ass is gone. I'm just letting you know cuz you're his brother. He's got fuckin' problems and I don't have the time to fuck with him." Samuel kept shaking his head in disappointment.

I raised my eyebrows helplessly, "Well, how about Donny? How's he doing?" I asked because I figured he would have major problems with anyone. Samuel was never the patient type.

Samuel shrugged, "Eh, he's lazy too. He just wants to sit around the shop, smoke weed, and play video games. But at least he's not addicted to pills."

Yep, he's got problems with Donny, too. I immediately knew that Alex was his current hatred target, and once Alex was gone Donny would be next in that spotlight. I was his hatred target at one point, even though he was the one who abused me – he always had to have a hatred target to function. Granted, if Alex was addicted to pills, that was a legitimate problem that needed to be addressed. Samuel didn't appear to have Alex's best interest at heart though.

I realized I was staring out the window in thought and shook my head, "Well, that's not good if Alex is addicted to pills. Where is he even getting them from?" I gave Samuel a questioning look.

Samuel stopped at a stoplight and turned his head to me, "Where the fuck do you think?"

Oh no, was Alex stealing pills from Samuel? Samuel was a loose cannon and dangerous. Alex was being an idiot and playing with fire. I suddenly appreciated Samuel coming to me and not beating the shit out of Alex, even if he was being abrasive about it. I suddenly agreed that Alex needed to not be around Samuel.

I reached my hands up behind my head and grabbed the headrest of the seat I was in, "Ok..." I leaned my head back against the headrest, "So, Alex needs to go back to Indiana. When does this need to happen?"

Samuel raised a hand to point downward dramatically, "Right fuckin' now. I'm drivin' him up this weekend."

"Ok, well, can I do anything to help?" I asked.

Samuel shook his head, eyes fixed on the road. "He just has a few bags of stuff. Just wanted you to know he won't be down here for long, so spend some time with him."

"Well," I inhaled with finality, hoping to bring the conversation to an end and go back home, "I gotta get back and get started on dinner, so can y-" I was interrupted.

"Bullshit, I know you ain't got a goddamn thing to do. We ain't done." He still sounded agitated.

Great... what else is there? Anxiety started setting back in as I noticed we were still driving further away from the apartments. Whatever distance we cover, we'll have to cover that same distance to get back. Ugh. I stayed silent and looked out the window. Anything I said now in protest, he would just argue with. Then things would escalate, he would start yelling at me, I would start crying, he would berate me further, and we would accomplish nothing. It was a stalemate, and since he was driving, I was not in control. Just let him say whatever it is he felt like he needed to get off his chest and get home without incident. That was my new goal.

"You know, I tried. I fuckin' tried." Samuel started, "I tried with all 4 of y'all mother fuckers. I feed you, I give you weed, I provide opportunity..." Samuel was raising his tone of voice and pointing at himself. "I'm trying to build something here for our family and nobody is helping!"

I inhaled deeply. I knew his game. He was playing the misunderstood savior again because his manipulation tactics weren't working out like he thought they should. "Man, look, you're the one who lured them down with dreams of becoming the next godfather and gave them access to copious amounts of weed. You expect them to just figure out how to run a business? They're looking to you for leadership. You gotta show 'em how it's done, man. Give them a good example."

Samuel rolled his eyes, "Lured? I'm not a fuckin' predator, Len."

I scrunched my eyebrows in doubt. "You're the one who sold them on this idea, this dream, of running a hydro shop. I don't know if you just have something to prove to my parents or if you just hate them, but you're the one who pushed so hard for this."

Silence hung in the air for a minute.

Samuel turned his head toward me, "You know," his voice sounded determined, "What was so bad with me that I had to go? Why did you accuse me of rape to your parents?" I could tell by the way he said the word 'rape' he was mocking me.

Ohhhh boy... This sucks, and I could feel my own emotions starting to churn beyond my control. I inhaled, "What the hell else would you call that? I was asleep and you did whatever the fuck you wanted. I didn't want our friendship to get sexual. I didn't want that. I didn't want any of that, but you never asked what I wanted."

Samuel slapped the steering wheel in frustration, "You had a fuckin' boner! You came! You enjoyed it!"

My heart wrenched. I hated thinking about or reliving that moment and here it was. "I was 13 and had morning wood. I came because that's how that fucking works. It's purely mechanical in nature and I couldn't stop it. I've felt guilty about all the orgasms for those 2 years that shit went on. You know I almost killed myself in your bathroom one night?" The emotions were bubbling over, and my lip had started to quiver.

"Bullshit!" He yelled at me. "You took my weed for years, all those gifts I bought you throughout the years, you loved every bit of it!" He made sure to remind me of the narrative he wanted me to believe.

That was one of his tactics. He would tell you how you felt and argue with you if you said otherwise. I had started crying fully now. It was ugly and I was sobbing. My heart was racing, and I was focusing 100% on trying to breathe and control my emotions. Bullshit? What a dick move but what else did I expect?

"Man..." I sobbed, trying my hardest to regain my composure, "I... I need to g- to go... home. I don't wa- wanna do this... right n- now." I was sobbing and my breathing had started doing the uncontrolled heaving thing while I was trying to talk. This was absolutely miserable and I only had myself to blame for getting into the truck in the first place.

"Nope." He sounded angry. "You always pull this bullshit. You break down in tears and shut down. I'm not letting you do it this time. We'll get back home when we get back home. Now answer my question!" Samuel's voice was as loud as it could get without yelling, but cracked with emotion near the end.

Suddenly, the entire situation with Uncle William was brought to the top of my mind as well. That was the same question I was hung up on with Uncle William. But this was different. It was obvious why I had to remove Samuel from my life. He took what he wanted from me and treated me like this if I protested. I knew he was going to argue with whatever I said and didn't have the emotional stamina for it, so I began to shut down on him, just like he said. I hated being predictable, but we knew each other well. This is how our conversations always go, and I don't know what ever gives me the idea it could be otherwise.

Samuel yelled and hollered, and eventually dropped me off at home, but the rest of the ride was all echoes and white noise to me. I don't remember anything else he said. Nothing could be louder than my emotions.

When he dropped me off, I was an absolute mess, emotionally. I went straight back to my room and laid down. I was extremely tired after that madness. But laying there on my bed, I thought of a question for myself: "You were free of him for 10 years. Why did you get back in contact with him in the first place?"

Why did I? That was an excellent question, and I honestly wasn't sure what the answer was. I tried to remember that decision. Oh right, that was back when I used Facebook...

It was right after I lost the first 75 pounds from running. I was feeling good and was scrolling through people I knew on Facebook. Was I searching for something? I think so, but I didn't know what. Adventure? Was I just feeling good after losing all the weight? Who knows what possessed me.

Alice... as I scrolled across that name, a big smile wrapped around my face. That was who I lost my virginity to at 16. I wondered how she was doing and hoped she was doing well. So I messaged her. If only the current me could go back to the moment of this memory and slap the hell out of myself...

Alice and I talked, just catching up with each other over the last 10 years before she convinced me to message Samuel. Why didn't I know better? What the hell was I thinking? It was all fuzzy and hard to remember. Keep thinking...

Oh right, it was an emotional choice that I made flippantly, without any thought given to my choices or to the consequences. Naively, I thought, 'We *started out as good friends. I wonder if we could find that place again and build something different this time. Maybe I could find some closure and forgive him, and good things could come of it.'* After all, I did care about him as a brother before things went sideways with us. That care was still in there somewhere.

But my emotional fairy-tale thinking was not based in reality. Why couldn't I see that then? Why, only after it was too late to avoid, was I forced to admit that things would likely never be different between Samuel and me. And now, my brothers were wrapped up in his hydro shop.

Laying there in my bed at JP and Ingram's place, I had a moment of clarity. Not once had my brothers hit me up to hang out while I was up there. I had asked to go to lunch with them a couple of times, but since Samuel managed their money and didn't actually give them paychecks, it all depended on him being there so he could pay. He insisted he pay for their lunches because they worked for him. He managed everything for them, so they would need his 'permission' to go do anything. He was their boss, their landlord, and their ride. I suddenly realized that he had set himself up in such a position that I had to go through him to access my brothers. Everyone did. And they had to go through him to access the outside world. He bought them video games and gave them weed to keep them there, paid for their food, didn't charge rent, just demanded labor and his permission to do anything.

I tossed in my bed, still sobbing quietly. The twins were not in a good position. And I had a sneaking suspicion that he might be trying to turn them against me behind my back by saying whatever he wanted. I had no proof, just a suspicion since California because Donny has been so distant and disconnected from me since then. I felt to blame for everything because I introduced Samuel back into my life. He influenced my brothers and it's all been drama and poor decisions since then. I had to stop whatever was happening, get my shit together, be a bastion for my brothers, and provide them with an exit ramp from that lifestyle.

Whatever funk I've been in since I got back home from California had gotten deep, probably depression or something, but I still had choices to make. Choices every day that could either put me in a better or worse place tomorrow. I'd been making poor decisions every day for the last few years, and it was catching up with me, compounding in effect. I knew I needed to make better choices, and I felt lucky for this moment of clarity. I couldn't count on this level of clarity all the time. My emotions were usually the loudest thing in my mind and they would steer my actions. I had to change something.

I tossed on my bed again, wiping more tears away. Alex was going back to Indiana, so that was good. Well, not really good at all. He'd be back with his group of friends that were into any drug they could get their hands on. But when we removed him from that environment, he started stealing pills in the new environment. Alex was going to need a lot of work, but I had to get my own shit together first before I could really help him at all. At least he would be away from Memphis. I could move him down to MS with me later after I got back on my own 2 feet if he could stay out of trouble until then.

The first step was fixing my marriage and moving back home. I rolled over in my bed, reached into my backpack beside my bed table, and pulled out a stuffed ladybug. It was only about the size of a really large coin and would completely fit in the palm of my hand. It was Liz's, and she had given it to me before I went to San Diego. I rubbed it and closed my eyes.

"Here, take this with you!" Liz bounced back to our room and rifled through her bedside drawers. She came back waving a small black and red object and set it against my chest with the most gorgeous smile.

"What's this?" I asked, grabbing and inspecting it.

Liz took a step back "That," she pointed at the small, round stuffed animal in my hands, "is my 'good luck ladybug'! I want you to take it with you to California and when you start to miss me, just pull it out and know that I love you and I can't wait to see you."

I looked up from the ladybug with the dumbest, hugest grin on my face and looked into her eyes, "I love this. This... this makes me incredibly happy. I love you. I would be honored to take your ladybug to California with me. It'll be good company until you get out there to take over the job." I smiled and kissed her.

I rubbed the stuffed ladybug again, continuing to remember all the things I love and miss about Liz. I tossed and turned in my bed and started crying pretty hard between memories, but eventually passed out with the ladybug on my chest.

Chapter 7

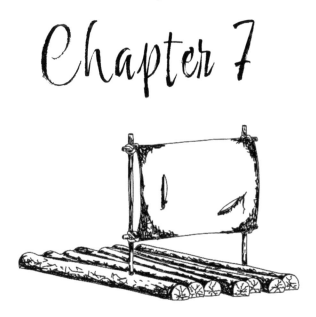

When I woke up the next morning, I felt groggy. Almost like I was really drunk or high the night before, but I was pretty sober. Was it all the crying? Ugh, who knows... I rolled out of bed.

I did my normal morning routine and saw Ingram and JP off to work with coffee and fresh smoothies. As I started cleaning for that day, everything felt different. Before, it felt like I was doing this for my own benefit and almost felt Buddhistic in purpose. Today, it felt like a waste of time. My purpose had shifted, and I knew it.

Why did it seem to take that emotional event to birth this new commitment? Maybe it was just the news of Alex being deported back to Indiana, but the emotions got pretty wild for me too. Maybe I shouldn't question it too much and just focus on making the most of it...

I decided to take Chester, JP's black lab, for a walk. I'd taken over doing that since I'd been there and spoiled him. I took him out for a short walk and potty break every time I had a cigarette or went for a run.

Walking around the apartment complex with Chester that day almost felt like saying goodbye to this place. Everything internally was leaning away from this and back toward home. I walked past the tennis court where I hurt my ankle, past the pool where we had many community parties, and past that drunk lady's place.

On the way back to the apartment, I knew I had to talk to Liz ASAP. I pulled out my phone and threw her a text, "Hey you, whatcha doin? You working today?"

I immediately got a reply back, "Nope, what's up?"

I did a little fist pump in the air and replied, "Got a minute to talk?"

"Of course!" She replied immediately again.

So I hit the shortcut to call her from the text screen as I was getting back to the apartment.

"Helloooooooo..." She answered, sounding silly.

I chuckled, "Hey you." I couldn't have been happier to talk to her then. I had a feeling she was going to want me to come back home, but I didn't want to assume anything. "I think I want to come back home, if you want me to come back." I swallowed the lump in my throat.

A moment of silence passed before I heard a little sniffle, "Of course... I want you back home." Liz was fighting some emotions too.

I couldn't speak for a moment I was so happy. "I honestly don't ever want to be away from you again if I can help it. I've been struggling and trying to figure it out since California, but I have to do something and move on with life and I can't see doing that without you."

"Whe-" Liz stopped to clear her throat, "When do you want to come back?" Liz asked, sniffling and trying to get her emotions under control.

I realized I had been standing in the living room with Chester still on the leash this whole time, "Honestly, as soon as possible. I don't have much in the way of plans yet, but I figure I can get someone who owns a truck to help me drive my stuff down. I don't have much here, so it'll be just one single quick trip." I took the leash off Chester's collar and put it up before heading back to my room.

"Will everything fit in the Neon?" She asked.

I sat down on my bed and thought about it for a minute. I looked around my room, thinking of where each of my things could fit. "Actually, I think so... If we put my computer in the trunk, the back seat should have enough room for my luggage and pillows..." I continued to think of logistics.

"Then I'll come down and get you on my next day off." Her voice was resolute.

I smiled and laid back on my bed, "I'd love that. How long do I have to get everything packed?"

Two days later, Liz pulled up to JP and Ingram's apartment complex in an empty Dodge Neon. I carried all my things out to the car and was done loading it up in 15 minutes.

When I came back inside from loading my things up, Ingram was standing about 5 feet away holding a fresh bowl. "Wanna smoke a 'see-ya-later' bowl?" He was grinning and holding it out for me.

I reached out to grab the bowl from him, "Of course! Thanks, haha!" I laughed and sat down on the couch next to Liz.

JP and Ingram sat on a second couch next to us and I passed the bowl after taking a hit, "You guys have been awesome. I'm glad to be going home now, but I really needed the time I've spent up here. You guys have provided that, and I couldn't be more thankful to have friends like you guys. I love y'all. Y'all better come play ESO with me." I reached two spread-out fingers up to my eyes and then turned my wrist to point those same two fingers at them on the opposing couch and smiled.

JP grabbed the bowl with a chuckle, "Well, we have enjoyed having you here. By far, you're the best roommate we've ever had. Nobody's ever cleaned up the house and made dinners before. We're going to miss you, but we're also going to miss that, hahaha."

Ingram raised both of his arms in the air, "I second that! Hahaha!"

JP offered the bowl to Liz, but she politely refused, "Nooooo, thanks, but I'm good. If I were at home and had gummies, it'd be a different story though." She smiled politely and sat up straight.

Ingram sprang up from the couch and disappeared down the hall. From the end of the hallway, we could hear his distant voice begin, "I found 2 unopened packages of THC gummies in an apartment today." We could hear his voice start moving back toward us, "Why the hell would you move and leave a bunch of shit like this behind? Anyway..." He handed Liz a sealed gummy package and sat on the couch. "Here, you take one. I didn't know you preferred the edibles." He grabbed the bowl and hit it.

Her eyes lit up, "Oooohhh... This is nice." She inspected the packaging. "So... they just moved and left this stuff behind?"

Ingram nodded, holding a lungful of smoke in.

I took the bowl from Ingram and looked at it. It was getting cashed, so I set it on the table, "I'm good on the bowl. We gotta get headed down so I can get unpacked before it gets dark, but you guys are coming down for my birthday in a few months, right?" I stood up, smiled, and opened my arms for a hug.

JP moved in for a hug first, "Of course. You let us know when to be there, and we'll be there."

Ingram hugged me, "You take it easy, Len. It's been really nice having you here and getting to know you."

I gave my hugs, turned around, grabbed Liz's hand, and we walked out to the car together.

We got home, I got my computer set up, unpacked all my clothes, and put my luggage away. Moby was excited to see me, so I played with him for a minute. I missed him, too. I eventually went to lay down on the bed next to Liz. I grabbed her hand.

"I love you." Our fingers now interlocked, I moved her hand to my lips and kissed the back of it. "I'm so very glad to be home. I need to focus on getting a job, but hopefully, this is the first of many good steps in the right direction."

Liz snuggled up to me, resting her head on my shoulder and wrapping my arm around herself. "I love you too. I'm so happy you're back. This winter was so cold and lonely."

I tightened my embrace on her and kissed the top of her head, "I will never spend another night away from you by choice ever again. I think it was ultimately a good thing for us to have split up for a little while, but I'm so happy to be back here with you."

"Yeah..." She moved her head around, using my shoulder to massage the back of her head, "... we got married so young. We barely knew ourselves, let alone each other. It was good, but I don't ever want to do that again."

I nodded quickly and emphatically, "Agreed! I don't want to do that again, either. Ever. We really did get married young, didn't we? We were, what? Barely 21? But it worked out because I knew everything, huh?" I joked.

Liz chuckled, "You certainly thought you knew everything." She stopped to look at me with a funny look on her face, "Still do, I'm afraid." She cackled and set her head back on my shoulder.

A big, dumb grin spread across my face, and I blushed a little, "Yeah, but I really do know everything now." I winked at her but couldn't suppress a ridiculous laugh. After a moment of laughter, we settled back down.

I started running my fingers through her long hair, "I'll start looking for jobs tomorrow. At bare minimum, I'll put in one application a day. More if I have the opportunity, but no less than one per day as a matter of principle." I reassured Liz that I was taking this seriously.

"Good..." she responded, quiet and motionless. I could tell she was getting tired, and it was getting late, so we crawled under the covers and passed out.

She was up at 3:30 the next morning for work. I woke up closer to 7, so she was long gone by the time I got up. I made some coffee, got a shower, and started browsing job listings on my computer for any job website I could find. I browsed and submitted applications, finishing cup after cup of coffee while doing so.

I had intended to clean up but got busy with filling out the applications. It was only noon, so I had plenty of time to clean up. I had to focus manically on seeding my application to every business in the North MS area.

It was then, after having spent the last 5 hours filling out applications, that I noticed something: this renewed commitment to get my shit together had me so focused that I didn't have time to be depressed or anxious. I had kind of... forgotten about it almost? Was this finally the depression loosening its grip? I had no clue, but was thankful, nonetheless.

I put my hands behind my head and leaned back in my computer chair, lost in thought. Where did this desire to get back on track come from? Where did the clarity of thought come from? Where did the confidence come from? I hated feeling like a slave to my emotions, but they get so intense sometimes that the only reasonable option seems like appeasing them in spite of any consequences to my life. Why did it seem like my emotions could change directions at any moment, seemingly outside of my control?

Was it Alex doing poorly which made me realize I had to get my life together if I wanted to be able to help him? Did I just hit a certain point of loneliness without Liz? Or were chemical reactions in my brain responsible for it all? Now, maybe I watched The Matrix too much as a teenager, but I refuse to believe anything can take my choice away from me. Sure, some things can have an influence on my choices, but it never sat well with me to use 'brain chemistry' as an excuse for my poor behavior.

Was it anything I did that helped me tap into this state of clarity and resolve? If so, what was it and how could I harness that to keep the debilitating emotions at bay? My head spun. I had no clue. I didn't even know how to look for a clue.

Searching my emotions like this always made me feel like I was lost at sea in the pitch black of the darkest night, unable to tell direction or gain any sense of awareness to navigate through the rough open waters. On a crappy raft made of nothing but planks and twine, I bob up and down helplessly as governed by the sea of my emotions. I go where the emotional sea pushes me. How the hell was I supposed to navigate that? It felt like other people in my life around me had speedboats or yachts and were just cruising through life.

But that's how it always feels, right? Each of us feels like we're the only one who is ill-equipped to deal with themselves, but surely that's a common human experience. Everything always seems like it's easier for others when we compare ourselves to those around us. I had to remind myself that I was no exception to this and that if other people can successfully manage their mental health and make good choices, then I can too, no excuses.

I felt good though, like I was inspecting a past event and not trying to figure out a solution to a presently persisting issue. Why did the depression 'feel' like it was over? The longer I sat in thought, the more questions I ended up with. Why does understanding yourself end up being such a huge challenge?

Just then, Liz came in the back door and surprised me. "I'm hoooooooooome!" She said in a silly voice.

I nearly jumped out of my computer chair.

Liz set her work bag down on the bar stool at the kitchen island counter and walked toward the living room where I was, "Hah! Did I scare you?" She added a little bit of sass with a raised eyebrow and pointed a finger at me.

I got up from my chair, "Maybe..." I smirked. "How was your day?" I started toward her in the kitchen.

Liz raised her chin, like proper royalty, "Today was a rather excellent day, Mister Kester." She nodded politely in Victorian fashion before smiling and reaching out to me for a hug.

I adjusted my glasses studiously, "Excellent, you say?" I met her embrace and kissed the top of her head, "Do tell, my lady."

Liz grabbed my outstretched elbow and I escorted her to the couch, "Ok, I'm done being proper, haha." She laughed and loosened up. "I may be the next manager of my store soon…"

I started to sit, but immediately stood back up in excitement and surprise, "Woah! That's huge! When is this happening?"

Liz inhaled and widened her eyes dramatically, "Well… you see… our current manager announced today that he is leaving the store for another position in the company in another part of the country. He pulled me aside after he announced it to the store and told me that I was his only recommendation to replace him as manager." She held her mouth open in awe and shook her head in wonder.

I sat down, "Woah, the only pick? So, you've pretty much got it, right?" I set my hand on her knee.

Liz bounced a little in her seat, "Okay, no, not quite. There still has to be a job opening posted to the job board for so many days, and anyone in the company can apply during that time. Then they'll interview everyone who applied and choose the one they feel best about like normal. Buuuuut…" She dragged the word out in dramatic fashion, "I'm the only one with the personal stamp of approval from the current acting manager, which I hope means a lot."

I nodded, "I see, I see. Still though, that's really good news! You're awesome babe. I love you." I looked at her with a smile and admiration. Liz was one of those people that looked to me like she was sailing the sea of her emotions with a speedboat. It at least looked from the outside like she was smashing victory after victory, while I kept getting stuck going in circles. But this isn't about me, and I had to remind myself of that. This is a happy moment for her and us, and I'm getting jealous. Where did those thoughts come from? I shook my head.

I made dinner and we watched some Walking Dead. Things felt right. I couldn't explain why, but I was just glad to feel good instead of bad for a change. I'd hoped this feeling would last.

But after many weeks of putting in applications and hearing nothing back in return, I started slipping back into depression. I'd gotten to the point where

I only put in one application per day, and sometimes it wasn't even realistic. It had become a box I needed to check on my daily routine, but why was I doing it if it hadn't produced any results? I quit putting in applications altogether after about 6 weeks. I started to wonder if maybe I was defective, and it showed through my resume somehow. I changed it often.

I started having problems sleeping, too. I would go to bed at a reasonable hour, like 10PM, and lay awake until 4 or 5AM frequently. Some nights I would get back up and play ESO. Some nights I would lay there in the silent darkness for hours. Sometimes though, it was really bad...

I sniffed, hoping not to wake Liz up with my crying. I had been lying in bed for 4 hours in pitch-black quiet and couldn't fall asleep. The problem was my brain. It wouldn't shut off. My brain would bounce from one guilty topic to another, torturing me with both past and present examples of my shortcomings. Why couldn't I have cool ideas that needed to be written down? Why was it always the same track of guilt that played in the background of my mind?

I wiped the tears from my eyes and ears and sat up slowly. I desperately needed to blow my nose. The crying reached a point of non-containment, so it was time to go cry somewhere that I wouldn't wake Liz up in the process. This was the second night in a row that I haven't been able to sleep at all, and it was looking like sleep wouldn't be back around until tomorrow night, if at all. I poured some water and sat down at my computer chair. So... what was I gonna do now?

I launched a video game, got to the main menu, and let it sit there for a minute. I sipped on my water in the silence and stared at the menu options. Nothing looked good, so I closed the game.

I launched another, closed it, then launched another and closed it too. I inhaled deeply and exhaled slowly. "Being human sure is fun sometimes." The thought made me chuckle a little bit. I took another sip of water and set it on the desk before opening Word. I wanted to put myself in the shoes of someone who had a completely different, wildly different, set of problems than I did.

'A Predator in his Prime' I typed out the title of the short story I had cooking up. I found another groove outside of poetry that morning. I wrote until Liz woke up and then made us some coffee. I saw her off to work and sat back down to finish writing. I got totally lost in the story.

I finished writing a few hours later and was exhausted. I decided to try sleeping again, even though it was now a little after 8 in the morning. Something inside, like a knot, released during the writing process, and I felt like I might actually be able to fall asleep.

Chapter 8

When I woke up, Liz was already asleep beside me. Holy crap... what year is it... I grabbed my phone to look at the time. The phone's light clicked on, and I could see 10:06 PM in big font across the middle of the screen. Damn...

I got up, habitually started a pot of coffee, and sat down at my computer. I had finished that story, so I'd have to start another. I wanted to start writing another story when I reminded myself it's been a while since I put any job applications in.

I reluctantly pulled up the job search page and noticed a listing for a Tier 1 IT job. Tier 1 is basic PC troubleshooting, and I knew how to do that very well. I could do that job in my sleep, so there was no reason not to apply. I sent my application in and, only after hitting the send button, did I wish I would have reviewed it at least once for errors. Oh well, I tiredly thought. I put an application out, so I can feel good about that.

I launched ESO and was surprised to find the majority of my guild mates online and playing. I joined them and we PvP'd until the sun came up, and then some. One or two people would drop and go to bed, and we'd pick up another one or two people who had just logged in. The group stayed roughly the same size the whole time.

I pushed my PTT key to transmit through Discord, "No other game can I rack up 600 kills in a night." I said. "I love this game and I hope it never changes. Anyway, I gotta get busy with some chores though, so I'll talk to you guys later."

I got an echo of goodbyes through my headphones and disconnected from the voice chat. I took my headphones off, set them on their rack, then got up & headed for the kitchen.

I was about half-way through running my dishwater when I got a call. I almost ignored it until I remembered I was giving that phone number to possible employers.

I dropped the forks I was holding and bolted to my phone across the kitchen.

"Hello? This is Len." Did I answer it in time, or had they already hung up? I waited for a reply.

"Hello, yes, Len Kester? This is Eli with Excel Technologies. I see you filled out an application last night just a couple hours after we posted the position. Are you still interested?"

Wow, they already called me back... I was stunned. I expected this one to turn out just like all the other probably hundreds of job applications I had put in by now, but here I was on this call. "Yeah, absolutely!" I answered back enthusiastically.

"I'm excited to hear that. You want to come in for an interview sometime this week? When is good for you?" Eli asked.

Uh... what day was it now even? I had to pull up a calendar, "Of course, let me double check my schedule... and make sure..." I was buying time so I could open the calendar, "I don't have anything... conflicting... that I may have... forgotten about..." Ok, today is Thursday, so I don't have much time left this week. "Oh yes, it's mostly clear this week. I can also move a couple things around if needed." I was staring at a blank-ass calendar, pretending to be busy. Why though?

"Are you good today or tomorrow?" Eli paused. "We're wanting to get this position filled as quickly as we can."

"I might be able to do it later today, but it would be a Hail Mary. I'll make some calls and see what I can do when we get off the phone, but let's plan on tomorrow for now."

"Perfect!" Eli sounded legitimately excited. "Let's meet at 9 AM tomorrow at our office here. Do you know how to get here?"

I thought for a moment, "Yeah, I have the address and can just punch it in to Google Maps."

"Perfect, Len. See you then!" Eli's tone of voice still sounded excited and positive.

"Thanks, talk to you later Eli!" I realized I may have sounded over-enthusiastic, but I didn't care. I was exploding with excitement. I finally got an interview. And not just any interview, one I was okay with and knew a lot about already. I wasn't going to need extensive training or anything. I honestly felt like I had a good shot at this one.

I immediately texted Liz, "I GOT AN INTERVIEWW!!!!!!! :D :D :D"

A few moments later, my phone chimed with a response message from her, "That's great! When?"

My fingers scurried excitedly and clumsily across the digital keyboard on my phone, "tmorrw, unles youll be homee erly enugh to run me down there tonighht." I hit send before I looked at the hot garbage I just typed out. Eugh… whoops. Calm down, Len…

Bzzt bzzt in my hands, "If they don't close ridiculously early, I'll be off in an hour and can take you then."

I inhaled in hesitation but stopped myself from thinking too much about it. My thumbs clicked the screen furiously, "Ok, let's do it tonight. That's enough time for me to get a shower and find something decent to wear."

I immediately called the number back that Eli called me from, "Excel Technologies, this is Eli…" he answered.

"Hey Eli, this is Len. I think I got a solution worked up that'll let me be down there in about an hour if you've still got time open today for the interview." I tried to control my excited breathing.

"Oh hey, Len," Eli replied optimistically, "I sure do. I'll slot you in for 1PM this afternoon. Sound good?"

"Absolutely!" I replied, "I'll see you then! Thanks!" That enthusiasm was bubbling over and making me self-conscious.

"Thanks Len!" He said and we hung up.

I looked down at my keyboard, "Don't fuck this up, Len." I told myself out loud before I took a shower and found some nice clothes. I ended up settling on some nice boot-cut jeans and a white button-up collared shirt with the sleeves rolled up and the top button loosened. I finished the ensemble with my black and white Converse with the black and white checker shoelaces.

After Liz got home, I drove into town, found the place, and parked out front. I gave myself one final glance-over to make sure I didn't have food or hair on my shirt, inhaled for stability, and headed into the shop.

Once I walked inside, I was greeted by a crazy man with an energy drink in his hand. "Heyyyyy! Are you Len?" He held one hand up in the air. Was he wanting a high-five? Was he celebrating my arrival?

"Hey, yeah, I'm Len. Is Eli around? I've got an interview with him shortly." I announced.

"Thaaaaat's me!" The hand without the energy drink in it pointed a thumb at himself. He was a middle-aged man, of average height, plump, with a goatee and short brown hair. He waved his hand and turned, "Come on back to the new conference room, oooooooooohh!".

I smiled; this is zany. There is no way this is the same guy I talked to on the phone who sounded professional. But it sounded fun, so let's see what this is all about. I stared at Eli's Hawaiian shirt he was wearing and followed him back to the conference room. When we got in there, I noticed one other person waiting. He was an older man, with grey hair, balding, but had piercing blue eyes. He was fit for a man his age and dressed nicely. He looked like a boss, too.

As we entered the room, the older man stood and Eli introduced him, "This is Dale," Eli held out one hand toward Dale and slammed the energy drink with the other. After swallowing, Eli continued "Think of Dale like... an office manager. Basically, anything he says goes. We work together as managers. My brother started Excel in another city and I run this office here. Dale helps me do that."

Dale reached toward me for a handshake. He was dressed in Khaki slacks, neatly pressed, and a button-up white-collared blue dress shirt. Over that, he wore a thin light-brown jacket made of a semi-shiny fabric of some sort. It looked fancy.

I met Dale's handshake with a smile and a nod, and we all sat down.

Eli crumpled up the empty energy drink can and threw it at a garbage can in the corner of the room and missed, "Damn." He shook his head and gave me a goofy look, "So what do you think?" He asked.

I nodded, thinking. After a moment, I started, "Yeah, I think it all sounds pretty straightforward. I can run the new store front you plan on opening and be the guy that stays here at the office fixing the computers that make it back here. If that's the expectation, I can handle that all day."

Dale smiled, unfolding his hands and reaching one across the table at me, "Then I think we'd like to offer you a position starting at thirteen dollars an hour if you think that's fair."

I was very surprised. I didn't expect to find out if I got the job for another week maybe. I didn't even think about the pay. I was instantly overcome with excitement, "Well, yes sir!" I returned the handshake, "When do you want me to start?" I stood up.

Dale stood up as well, "How does this coming Monday sound?"

It was Thursday now. They must have really needed someone. "I can make it happen." I answered confidently, unable to wipe the huge dumb grin off my face.

Eli reached out his hand to me, "It was good to meet you, Len. Looking forward to things. We'll see you this Monday morning!"

I returned the handshake, "Thank you. It was good to meet you guys as well. See y'all Monday!"

I walked out to the car feeling taller than any building in the country. To me, it wasn't just a job interview. It was the step I had been stalled for months on. I pulled out of the parking lot in our grey Neon and cranked the music.

"YEEEEAAAAAAH I WAS UP ABOVE IT!" I sang along to the lyrics and felt like a million bucks. Was it just because I was finally making progress? No, there was something else there too. These people, these complete strangers, trusted me enough to give me a chance. I could give myself a break now, knowing that I was good enough for a complete stranger to place their faith in me to complete a task. I was full of gratitude and good energy.

I pulled into my driveway way too fast, came to a quick stop, shut the car off in drive, put it back into park, manically wrestled the keys from their resting place in the steering column and rushed inside as fast as I could. My heart was racing.

I shut the door behind me, "AEAEAEAEAEAEAEAE!!" I excitedly screeched an unintelligible call of victory.

"Excuse me, Mr. Kester?" Liz said.

I could hear her footsteps getting closer, so I set my keys and phone down on the kitchen counter and waited beside the doorway I knew she would be coming through.

"IGOTDAJOB!" I said as quickly as I could and jumped at her when she came through the doorway.

"AHH!" She screamed in surprise. She was delightfully easy to scare. "Oh my... you..." She breathed and waggled a finger at me, "Did I hear that right? You got the job?"

I nodded excitedly, "It blew me away. I was not expecting to get hired on the spot like that. I was expecting to spend the next week or two waiting nervously for a job offer that may or may not ever come." I grabbed her shoulders and kissed her forehead, "I start Monday."

She grabbed my waist and pulled in for a hug, "I'm so happy for you." She nuzzled my shoulder, "Did you have to take a drug test?"

I shook my head, "Nope. Even though I've spent the last 3 months completely sober, apparently it wasn't required." I shrugged, "I'm not necessarily complaining, but I did think it was odd. They hired me in a hurry."

Liz looked up from my shoulder, at something behind me. "Uh... baby..." She pointed out the window.

I turned around and saw the driver's side door of the car left wide open. "Oh... whoops... I think I uh... I'll go get that..." I laughed.

We made dinner together and Liz had to go to bed immediately afterward to be up at 3:30 AM. But it was only 7:30 PM, so I decided to stay up. Normally, I'd have loaded up ESO and played online with my friends, but I didn't want to play tonight. I was going to start a new job on Monday, and I wanted to be sure I was as prepared as possible. But what could I do right now to prepare?

Hmm... I wondered. Nothing really. I put my headphones on and listened to some music. I looked up Alibi by Thirty Seconds to Mars, one of my favorite songs of theirs.

"No warning sign, no alibi... took our chance, crashed and burned... no we'll never ever learn... I fell apart. But got back up again... and then I fell apart, but got back up again, yeah." Jared Leto's voice rang in my ears and I let the emotion pour over me.

As the song played, I just sat there, captive, thinking about how many times I'd fallen apart over the years. I spun my chair around and looked at the back of my couch since my computer was set up in the front room. I remembered the time I leaned against the back of my parent's couch, fallen apart.

Teenage me cried uncontrollably, sitting on the floor and leaning against the back of the old couch. In my hands was Dad's revolver, which I had no clue how to use. I hadn't even checked if it was loaded, to be honest. But I sat there and really thought about whether I wanted to die. I wanted my problems to go away, but I didn't really want to die. I still wanted to learn so many things. And it took me being there at that point to realize that I wasn't really suicidal, I was just confused and didn't know how to get out of my situation.

I was letting Samuel sexually and emotionally abuse me, but he gave me all the weed I could ever want, and he was on my side in the battle against my parents. I thought he was the only person that would ever understand me. My parents didn't like anything I wanted to do as I was discovering who I was. I had to hide things from them and lie so I could go out with the friends they didn't want me to go out with. Mom tried to control everything. She dressed me for my first year of school in Memphis, and it went about as horribly as you'd imagine. She tried to force me into religion, and that went horribly, too.

Caught between an abusive situation and parents that were pushing me into religion, I wanted out from between all that pressure. And sitting behind my parent's couch that day with Dad's revolver in my hands, I wondered if that was the answer to my problems.

I spun back around in my computer chair, glad that I 'got back up' from that instance of 'falling down'. I continued to think about the situation I was in when that happened.

Samuel was on my side then... but he kind of helped create that conflict. Some conflict would have happened without him there, but he fanned the flames. He was totally seeking an opportunity to distance me from my parents. But why? I didn't know and I didn't want to think about why. He would seem to care sometimes, but then at other times, he would be an absolute ass and just criticize me relentlessly. Uninvited, he would psycho-analyze me and point out my deepest flaws, most of which were complete horseshit, but he thought he knew better than anyone else. He was really on his own side all along. And if I distanced myself from him again as I did as a teenager, I would also be distancing myself from my little brother, Donny.

I poked around my writings folder on my computer and pulled up the poem I wrote Uncle William. I thought about the depression I'd been stuck in since California, and it finally felt like that might be lifting. Did the depression decide to lift on its own, or was there something I'd done to influence the depression somehow? Was it my good choices in getting a job that helped, or did the depression fading help me to get a job? I really couldn't tell which was the cause and which was the effect.

I decided I'd attribute it to the good choices and move on with things. Maybe my problem was that I was too introspective. Maybe I needed to think less and do more... That sounded like an impossible task. My entire belief system about being the best human I can be is shaped around making better choices. I can't just blindly do without thinking about it... that's how I think we end up with the huge societal issues we have.

However, I could at least try to turn that volume down a little bit... maybe achieve something in the middle. A good balance... Uncle William's words rang in my ears, "Balance in all things, Len..." He told me that many times and that still seemed like solid advice, in spite of his current character. I knew it was important not to throw the baby out with the bathwater, as they say, so I tried to not let the good lessons go.

I leaned back in my chair and inhaled deeply. I wish I could figure myself out... It always feels like the solution is just out of reach and if I just keep pressing for answers, I'll figure something out that I hadn't seen before, and I'll finally make sense to myself. What did this idea of balance even look like concerning mental health?

I rubbed my temples and got up. I need to get some sleep and just focus on the work... Just focus on tomorrow...

Chapter 9

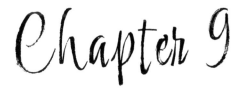

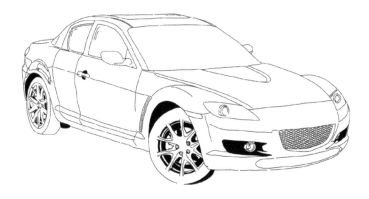

I tossed over in my bed and looked at the time, unable to sleep anymore. I picked up my phone and hit the volume button on the side so I could see the time. The light pierced the darkness of the room, and the time read 5:47... I had 13 minutes before my alarm went off. I'd been awake since I got back from dropping Liz off at work at 4:30. I tried to get back to sleep, but it was no use. I was way too focused on my first day of work coming up today.

Why was I still waiting for my alarm at this point? I convinced myself to just get up and get started with my day already. I did the usual morning routine, made coffee, took a shower, and got ready. I liked the business casual style, so I basically dressed the same as I did for the interview. Nice jeans, Converse Chucks, and a nice single-color button-up collared shirt. I'd roll the cuffs up by two full rolls on each arm. I removed my fake plug earrings and set them in our jewelry box in the bathroom cabinet. I needed to look professional.

I played with Moby until it was time for work. Moby was almost 2 years old now and he was a big buddy. He had long black fur and looked like a border collie/black lab/chow mix, or maybe a flat-coated retriever. His favorite toy was a thick, industrial rubber toy we called the "tugly". And he knew the word, too.

I slapped my thighs and crouched a little bit, "Where's your tugly at buddy?"

Moby barked once.

I raised my hands into the air, "Where is it?"

Moby barked again, ran around in a circle, and started sniffing around for the tugly. He ran into the other room and came back with it in his mouth. I reached for it and he immediately pulled away. Ok, he wants to play chase. I chased him around for about 10 minutes until I was a little winded.

I looked at my phone and it was still about 45 minutes before I needed to be at work. Ehh, I'll just head in early. I figured I'd take 30 minutes before the day starts to look around and see if I can fix any computers early. I was salary, so I knew my new employers wouldn't have a problem with overtime or anything.

I pulled up to the place and it was locked. I beat the owner here on my first day, so I felt pretty good about that at least. Dale was the first one to get there at around fifteen 'til 8, so I got out of the car and followed him up to the door.

I waved as I approached Dale, "Morning!" I said, making sure he saw me. I didn't want to scare my new boss on my first day there.

He waved back, "Well good morning! How long have you been waiting out here?"

I chuckled, "Oh just a few minutes. Not long. I figured I'd head in a little early and get familiar with things."

We approached the door together and Dale smiled wryly, "And you let a locked door stand in your way?"

I laughed, "Yeah, I guess I did. Fear of vandalism charges and all that."

He laughed and unlocked the door, "Well, the first order of business before anything else... and I mean -AN-Y-THING-" He enunciated each syllable of the word slowly and carefully, and paused to look at me with wide eyes, "Coffee!" He nodded and started laughing.

I joined in his laughter, "I couldn't support this effort more, sir." I said.

We made coffee and chit-chatted about tech, then he showed me the tech bench area, which had no computers currently in need of service, and then showed me the storefront they had just finished remodeling for me to setup like a retail store. This IT company was renting a space from the old mall, and so they just rented the next space down from their current space and expanded there.

Dale pointed at the wall, "Over here we're going to get some of that pegboard material up. And we've got a logo that will be ready to pick up in a couple days that we're gonna put over here." He pointed to another spot. "So, we've still got a few finishing touches to put on it, but it should be ready for you to setup in a few weeks. Until then..." He pointed at the door leading to the interior of the mall, "I'll show you what work we have for now." He opened the door and started walking across the open walkway to the store front across from us.

I followed Dale, looking around. I hadn't been in this mall much, since I thought it was nearly abandoned. "So, what are they doing with this mall? I see a lot of medical businesses in here, but nothing that I would expect to see in a mall except the food court down there." I pointed at the opposite end of the mall from us.

Dale sipped his fresh coffee, "Well, this place got bought out a few years ago and the owner has been slowly trying to turn this old mall into a medical complex. He's puttin' all kinds of money into this place."

I nodded in understanding, "Ahh, and we're his IT guys."

Dale turned around at me and winked, "And this place..." he pointed to the empty business space we were now standing in front of, "...is a new home healthcare provider who's moving in soon. We need to run all the ethernet cables for them and terminate the patch panel and all the outlets for them. Tyler will be here soon to help you get started. In the meantime, check out the mall. Walk around and take a look at all the renovations happening and new businesses moving in. We'll probably be running cable for each of the businesses that move in here. I'll be in my office if you need anything." And he turned and walked back over to our office, disappearing back into the unfinished storefront.

I ran nearly a half-mile of cable that first day, fishing the wires down through the walls to Tyler, who would mark each end with a unique number. My first day was 8 hours long and we went home. I was hired into a salary position, so I wouldn't get overtime. But I was also promised that they did try to keep the overtime to a minimum. Day 1 turned out to be true to that.

When I got off work, I had to go pick Liz up. She had been off work for a couple of hours already and had to wait at her store for me to come get her. I picked her up and we headed home.

Liz set her drink down next to her empty plate, "That was really good..."

I nodded, gulping a piece of barbecued chicken. I knew I had barbecue sauce all over my face, but I didn't care. "Oh my god... I don't know why I don't grill more often..." I said, setting the leg bone on my plate.

When I looked up at Liz, she was just shaking her head at me. "What? You don't like my barbecue beard? Come give me a kiss!" I puckered my lips at her and started making kissy noises.

Liz just looked at me and handed me a wet washcloth.

I grabbed the wet washcloth and chuckled, "You know what I always say..." I started wiping my face.

Liz nodded with a smile, "It's not truly good unless it makes a mess... Oh, trust me. I know."

"Thaaaaat's right!" I said, wiping the last bit of barbecue sauce from my face, "And this... was delicious." I put the washcloth down on the table. "You know, I should get my own car now. You having to wait 2 hours after work for me to come pick you up is no good and me having to wake up at 3:30 AM to take you to work is no good."

Liz grabbed her paper plate and threw it in the trash, "Yeah, I was thinking about that today. We've made things work with one car for almost 8 years now. I think it's time to become real adults and get two cars." She snorted out a chuckle.

"Hmmm..." I wondered out loud. "We could go tomorrow after work?"

I got off work the next day and hurried out to the car. I had been looking at cars and reviews all day, but still had no clue what I wanted. I picked up Liz and we headed to go look at a couple of different dealerships. We stopped at the first dealership, handled the wave of salesmen, and then browsed the lot. After not seeing anything good within my price range, we moved to the second dealership.

Walking up and down the rows, I realized everything that I liked was well out of my price range. As we toured this second lot, I came across a dark grey 2008 Mazda RX-8. It was love at first sight. The whole world faded and nothing but me and the car existed in a time bubble. I ran my hands along the contours of the front tire wells, the hood, the headlights... She was perfect. I was scared to look at the price tag because I didn't want this dream to be crushed, but I was pleasantly surprised when I did. It was almost $2k below my budget price! This was too good to be true. It had to be this RX-8. This was the one.

I took it for a test drive and fell even further in love. I didn't know what a rotary engine was, but it made the car ride feel so smooth... like you were flying a spaceship, not driving a car. I couldn't get over how different the experience was from a traditional piston engine. I was hooked. I didn't know it then, but I'd joined an international brotherhood of passionate rotary nerds that night.

I told Liz I was going to take the interstate home. She could follow me, but I was probably going to punch it as soon as I hit the interstate. I reserved any of that foolery during the test drive, but I really wanted to open it up and see what she could do now that she was mine.

I sat in the turn lane waiting for the light to turn green so I could turn onto the onramp for the interstate. I had done some reading while we were waiting on papers to transmit during the car sale, so I knew that this engine could achieve high RPM's easily and it was a good idea to hit high RPM's regularly to burn and blow out any excess carbon on the rotors so that the rotor seals could function properly. 'Drive it like you stole it.' One bit of advice read.

The light turned green, and I turned left. Once the car straightened out on the onramp, I punched it. The RX-8 isn't a crazy muscle car. Its draw isn't in the horsepower, the draw is in the smoothness of the ride and the insane handling. However, it still had some respectable power. I wasn't going to be winning drag races, but it was perfect for me. I hit the speed limit well before I entered the interstate, so that was sort of anti-climactic. But after driving the Neon for years, this thing was amazing to me. It felt so good to ride around in the RX-8. The turns felt like the car was glued to the road because the center of gravity was so low and perfectly centered.

The engine sounded like a muzzled lion with its factory exhaust, though. She needed to be allowed to roar. I had plans...

The next day, I pulled up to work in my stock RX-8 feeling like a million bucks. Dale and I were the first ones there again, and Dale immediately knew all about the RX-8 and the history of rotary engines. I even learned a few things from him and found out that he has a long history with sports cars.

Nobody else at work knew what it was and thought I had dropped $50k+

for it. It looked so good. Nobody could believe it was only $12k. I loved that car.

The following months were good months and went by quickly. I put my head down and worked. I began to pay debt off, had a new hobby in my car, and felt successful at my job. I could feel the depression lifting day by day, but I still had to make the choice to push through it each day - to get up and do what I decided I was going to do. It was hard until it became normal again, which took quite a few months.

I pulled into work and parked out front. I had started bringing my personal computer to work and setting it up on the counter in the store front. I had built it myself, so it had custom LED lights, a liquid cooling loop, and some nice hardware. I wanted to have something flashy in the shop to catch people's eye and draw some attention. It worked, but people would just come in and ask about the computer and then leave without buying anything.

I finished plugging all the peripherals into my computer and connected it to the overhead speaker system. Eli and Dale said they didn't care what I played, but I wanted to have something that didn't have any lyrics but was just good background music. So, I put on Juno Reactor. Their entire library of music was so vast, I could just put it on random and never hear the same song twice in a week.

I was busy checking local prices on the things we sell to see if anything needed to be price-adjusted when the door chime rang, and someone walked in the store.

"Hey! Welcome to Excel Technologies." I said, looking up at the visitor.

The visitor made eye contact with me, "Yo! Hold up... is that... is that Juno Reactor I hear?" He cocked his head and cupped his hand to his ear.

I smiled wryly, "You, sir, know good music." I reached out to him for a handshake across the front counter, "I'm Len."

He shook my hand, "I'm Jack. How long have you guys had this shop open?"

I turned and adjusted some cables on a shelf, "We've only been officially open for about two weeks now. It took us a couple of months to get the place finished, but we're finally open."

Jack looked outside the shop at the empty mall, "I bet you don't get a lot of traffic in here though, do you?"

I shook my head and started chuckling, "Nope. I had wondered about that, but I've just been asked to run it. I think it might be a better idea to have an internet café and partner up with the coffee shop down in the food court. But..." I chuckled again, "I do as I am told because those decisions are above my paygrade. So, what brings you here today?"

Jack leaned against the front counter, "Oh I'm just hangin' out today. I used to work here a few months ago but got another job. I come back sometimes to see Eli and Dale and everyone because they're still my friends. I haven't noticed you yet though, how long have you been with the company?"

"Heh..." I stifled a laugh, "A few months." I tried to keep from cracking a smile but failed entirely.

Jack immediately started laughing, too. We both knew I was his replacement.

We talked for a few hours that day. We had so much in common from our teenage years. We both pursued the same profession in computers, had a passion for video games, and shared so many interests. We immediately hit it off as friends and exchanged phone numbers.

I didn't realize how much I needed a local friend until Jack came around. We ended up having a lot in common. Both of us were raised in Christian conservative homes and had found our own paths away from that lifestyle. A lot of the folks our age who were our friends in high school were still mostly living at home with their parents, playing guitar, and smoking pot. Jack and I bonded over the fact that we chose to do things differently than most of our high school friends and our parents. We both valued independence and autonomy.

I drove my RX-8 home after work that night and appreciated how different my life was from just a few months ago. It was like a paradigm shift had occurred. I felt like I owed it all to my choices. It was uncomfortable, but if I hadn't made the choices I did, I wouldn't be where I am now. I was thankful but didn't feel like I understood everything that was happening inside my own skull. I wanted to believe that I had superseded depression with a clear understanding of life, but I honestly just felt like I got lucky somehow. I really didn't know what to attribute the change to.

I reminded myself not to think about it too much. I got home, made dinner, and watched a couple of movies with Liz before we called it a night.

Chapter 10

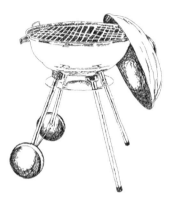

That following Thanksgiving, Mom and Dad came down to visit and brought my little brothers, Alex and Joseph, with them. Donny was still working with Samuel at the hydro shop, and he didn't really want to come down with us and spend time because Mom was there. Plus, Donny was allergic to cats, and I had two of them.

I was still so excited to have them down. This was exactly the opportunity that I had hoped to be able to create when I was living with JP and Ingram. I had worked myself into a position where I could now be of some real use to Alex and Joseph and help them get out of Indiana.

I stood in the hallway of the Excel office. Alex and Joseph stood on either side of me. I put one arm around each of my little brother's shoulders, "These little dudes are the most awesome little dudes on the face of the planet." I gave them both a squeeze. "And behind me are my Mom and Dad."

Dad stepped forward and shook all my co-workers' hands while Mom introduced herself and threatened to tell embarrassing stories about all of us.

I rolled my eyes, "Do your worst, Mom." I jostled my brothers with my arms and showed them the rest of the office. We headed back home after saying a round of goodbyes to everyone there.

When we got home, Dad cooked us some of his famous beer ribs.

I added one more bone to the growing pile now on my plate. "Those are perfect every time, Dad, I don't know how you do them so well, so consistently. I got lucky and made your level of steaks a couple of times, but I can't tell you why those perfections turned out like they did." I shook my head.

Dad laughed, "The key to the ribs is the 6 hours they spent in the oven, soaked in beer at two-hundred degrees. They only go over to the grill to get that char and caramelize the barbecue sauce." He winked. "That's it, man. That's all there is to it."

I raised a single finger in remembrance, "Oh wait, you do the same thing with steaks, right?"

Dad nodded, "Yep! I still do. I'll buy the big chuck roasts, cut them up into... you know..." he motioned with his fingers, "about two-inch-thick slices, marinade them in beer, cook them for a couple of hours at one-fifty, then finish them up on the grill with whatever seasonings you want. Mmmm..." He pinched his fingers together.

Mom stood up, "I'm gonna go lay down, okay?" she spoke to the table.

We all said "Okay," and waved her off. After all, she did spend most of her time laying down on the couch so none of us were surprised. After a few more minutes, Dad and Joseph went to bed too.

I looked at Alex, "Looks like it's just us. Come on, let's go back to the office and talk. I'm not tired."

Alex grinned his iconic smooth grin, "Aight, yeah. Me either."

I sat down with my legs crossed under me on the air mattress I had set up in the office for Alex, "So, how you doin' up there bud?" I looked at him sincerely.

He shrugged, "It's aight. Why?"

I made eye contact with him, "Bud, I just... I don't think there's a lot of opportunity up there in Indiana. Where you guys live, it's basically cornfields and drugs. Let's be real, you're no farmer so that only leaves one reason to stay up there. And I'm worried about your health if you go too far down that road."

He sat next to me and wrapped his arms around me, "Lenny, I love you. I hope you know that. All the shit that Uncle William and Samuel talked, it don't mean anything to me. I know they're bitter assholes. But I gotta be up there with my friends. Dustin just had a lil girl, and I gotta help take care of that lil girl. Dustin's into some bad shit. Besides, you remember how badly it went last time I stayed with you, right?" He looked at me with a straight face.

I shrugged, "I mean, yeah, I guess I can be kinda overbearing sometimes. I don't mean to do it to demean you by it, I just... I love you bud. I care so much and I want you to be happy and successful."

Alex tightened his hug around my chest and set his head on my shoulder, "It's not just you. Yeah, I had a hard time understanding you sometimes, but man, I'm broken and you don't gotta take care of me. You're too smart to waste it on me."

My eyebrows crumpled up and contorted with concern and confusion as I looked down at his head on my shoulder. "Buddy... that's so sad... what do you mean?" genuine surprise and confusion prevented me from saying anything intelligent.

He lifted his head to look at me, "No, like... I dunno. I respect you too much to ever let you put up with me like we put up with Mom. Don't worry about me, I'll be fine with Mom and Dad. Besides, Dad needs my help dealing with her crazy bitch ass."

I laughed, "Damn, you and Dad have bonded since the last time I was up there, eh?" I poked at his rib.

He released his hug and laid down beside me, "Yeah, a lil bit. We go fishing now. He's cool. He used to be *such* a huge douche though." He placed dramatic emphasis on the word 'such'.

I laughed again. "Yeah, he was a real hard-ass back in Memphis, wasn't he?"

He rolled his eyes, "Somethin' like that. He calmed down a lot since he retired though. Like, he can be pretty cool most of the time."

I shook my head, "Mom still sleeping all the time?"

He inhaled sharply, "Man, fuck that bitch. She don't do anything but sleep on the couch and bitch."

Oh boy... that's obviously a tender subject now. Maybe I should try to change the topic back to opportunity. "Fair enough. Anyway, look bud... think about it." I started. "I can get you a job working with me. I can train you how do everything we do there in just a few months. You're smart, too. You already know a lot of the basics, so that'll make it even easier for you. You'll catch on quickly; I know you will." Did that sound as desperate as it felt like it did?

Alex's face dropped, "Man, I don't know if I wanna do computer stuff. They piss me off. And people piss me off even more."

I nodded slowly, "Okay... well, what are your plans?"

He bobbed his head back up, "I dunno, I'll figure something out. I got time."

He was only 20, so he was right. He did have some time to figure things out. I didn't want to pressure him to have everything figured out at 20, but I was still worried that he wasn't really giving his future the forethought it deserved. I patted his leg, "You're right, Bubba. I just get excited because I want what's best for you. So, I see something that might be a good opportunity, and I get excited about it. I love you and I'd love to have you living down here with me. I think that would be hella fun." I smiled at him with all the compassion I could muster.

We went to bed shortly after that, but I couldn't sleep because I was thinking about that conversation. Was Alex telling me that he didn't want my help? Was I too late to do any good? The one thing that was certain was I couldn't do anything to help him if he didn't want what I was offering. It wasn't right to manipulate him into coming down, so I had to be okay with letting him make his choice to stay up in Indiana. I was heartbroken, but I still had Joseph to think about.

Joseph was still too young to get a job and move out on his own. He was only 15, so I had a few years to prepare as much as possible.

The next day was Saturday, so I invited Jack and his family over to meet my family.

"Ohhh, I think they're here!" Liz hollered out from the kitchen.

Dad was showing me some of his knives when I heard Liz call out. I jumped up, "Oh, be right back, Dad! Jack, Tiffany and Logan are here!" I excitedly rushed to the front door and opened it.

"Eeeyyyy!" Jack said, "Where's Papa Kester? I got a lil somethin' for him."

I smiled ear to ear. "He's back in the office. He was showing me some of the new knives he's gotten recently. C'mon, I'll get him to come out to the kitchen and we'll have a few beers."

I ran back, got Dad, and we came out to the kitchen together. "Dad, meet Jack." I motioned toward Jack. "And Jack, meet the man, the myth, the legend, my Dad himself." I motioned a hand toward Dad.

Jack shook Dad's hand, "Mr. Kester. Len told me so much about you. It's good to finally meet you. I, uh... brought you a gift." He got this shitty grin on his face and handed Dad a small cylindrical present wrapped in birthday wrapping paper.

Dad looked at Jack and grinned in response, "Ok, ok, let's just see what the Marine gets for the old Army Veteran." He chuckled sarcastically and started unwrapping the present, revealing a black T-shirt. He unrolled it and it said 'The Army: Because even marines need heroes sometimes'. Dad started laughing so hard. "Boy, I wasn't expecting that one. I'll have to find you a good T-shirt and give it to you next time I come down here." He held his beer up to Jack, "Salut, Marine! Where's your beer?" he said in full drill sergeant mode.

Jack laughed, "Oh you know, I just saw it and thought you might appreciate it." He grabbed a beer, opened it, and clinked cans with Dad.

They talked together for a minute before Dad took his old shirt off and put the new shirt on that Jack had just gotten him.

I shook my head and smiled, "And Jack, these are my little brothers, Alex and Joseph." I pointed at each of them respectively. "These little dudes are awesome."

Jack stepped up, "Well hey there, fellas. You guys have had to put up with this guy as your big brother?" He made a gross face and pointed at me.

Alex laughed, "Yeah, but he's aight sometimes." Alex looked at me with an assuring smirk.

Jack looked at Joseph, "So how many girlfriends you have?" He gave Joseph a wink.

Joseph blushed and looked at the ground, "None."

Dad made his famous BBQ chicken legs since I had bragged about them so much to Jack. Whatever he grilled always turned out perfect.

The only way I could have been prouder is if Donny were there too. We weren't a perfect family, but for better or worse, this was our family. And finally, it felt like a 'better' scenario and not a 'worse' scenario. We hadn't done any holidays as a family in years. I'm not even sure how life got too busy for that, but I'm glad we were together as a family again for this. I was so happy for the family to see that I was doing well after so long of not doing well. Nobody but Liz saw those bad days though, so they might not even know that there was a struggle there.

I sat out on my front porch alone that night. Everyone was asleep, but I was still worried about Alex. If only there was a way I could get him to stay here and never go back up to Indiana. He cared about the friends he had, and I understood that. I also understood that they were not a good group of people for his long-term health. How could I be supportive and be a good big brother if he's doing something I disagree with? I could only hope that rock bottom wouldn't be too bad for him and let him make his choice. But I had to be here and ready if he ever reached out.

I hung my head between my shoulders and lit a joint. That didn't feel like much of a solution, but how much control did I really have in Alex's life? All the power was in his hand to make a choice. I could only make that choice easier for him to make, but he still had to be the one to make it. I have to respect his choice above all else, right?

I inhaled a large toke and sat down in the dark at my front patio table. I looked out across the moonlit grass in the front yard. I remembered when Alex lived with me for a few months. I hadn't gone to California then. I was so young and I thought I knew everything... I was trying to push him to get his shit together, so to speak. The conversation happened right there near the front patio.

I waved my hand at Alex, "No bud, you're missing the point. You could get a job within walking distance of here. I'm not going to kick you out, you're welcome to be here as long as you like, but I do hope you get a job. And not even for rent. You need to be able to start building your life. Like, I don't want any of the money you make. It's all for you. But you need it so you can get a car and a place of your own eventually." I thought everyone was like me and valued independence.

Alex scoffed, "I'm 17, Len... you're acting like I'm 30 and still living in mom and dad's basement. Let me just do me... Jeez..." He pleaded in frustration.

I shook my head, not understanding where the disconnect was coming from, "No bud, I'm not saying that at all... I just think that you're not taking your future seriously enough. That's all. I mean, you're such an amazing artist. Why don't you find some way to utilize that? Be your own boss and make your own life that way. Living with Mom sucks, and I know it does."

Alex wagged his head back and forth in frustration, "Man, I love you, but this is too much. I don't want to fight with you about my lifestyle like I do with Mom and Dad. I like our relationship and I don't want to ruin it."

I stepped over to him and gave him a hug, "Buddy, I'm sorry... I don't mean anything bad by anything I say. I just... I really care. And I get really worried that..." I choked up and couldn't say the words that I wanted to, "Look, the only one who can take care of you like you deserve to be taken care of is you. I love you bud. I love you so much." I tightened my arms around him.

I leaned back in my chair, still observing the moonlit grass. I took another drag off the joint and held it in. Alex chose to leave my house and move back to Indiana after just a few short months back then. Had I not driven him away by being so demanding of what he does with his life, things might've been different now. I tried so hard to do right by him, but had I ended up doing him wrong somehow by accident? I shook my head, unsure where to place things.

I looked at my finger and remembered driving seven-year-old Alex to the emergency room.

"Ohhhhgggg..." I was getting nauseous in the backseat of my parent's minivan.

Alex giggled as he pulled his finger free from the towel. Blood was squirting from his finger. There was a little bit of meat and skin on the back of his ring finger, just above his fingernail cuticle near the joint. This little piece of meat and skin was the only thing keeping the top half-inch of his digit currently attached to the rest of his body. I had it neatly wrapped up in a towel and was actively applying pressure to it when he slipped his finger out.

I was white as a ghost, but also trying to catch the blood with the towel and get his finger back into the towel in one piece so the doctors could sew it back on.

Alex giggled, squirting blood at me.

I swallowed hard, breathing shallowly, "Buddy, you gotta stop..." I hated throwing up, so I would refuse to puke until my stomach gave me no choice. I just fought with nausea instead. "I really need you to let me put your finger back in this towel." I looked at the towel that was covered in blood now.

Dad stopped holding back his laughter, "Aw, it's just a little blood, son. You'll be fine."

Alex giggled again and I tightened my grip on the towel. "Are we close?" I asked between my shallow breathing.

Still staring at my finger, I stopped and re-lit the joint. My lighter lit up the patio where I was sitting. I love that little dude so much. I was afraid he was going to mess around until he felt like he was so far behind everyone else his age that he would feel no point in trying to catch up with anyone and possibly give up on life altogether like Mom had done. I didn't think Mom would give up on life and sleep it away on the couch, but it happened. If it happened once, it could happen again. But, I had to not project my fears onto him and just let him make his mistakes and be here for him when he's ready.

Most importantly though, I had to make sure I kept depression at bay. I had to grow my career and get more stable. If there was ever another opportunity to get Alex down here, I needed to be in the position to act on it when it happened.

I leaned forward in my chair, resting on my elbows and finishing the joint. But I really couldn't explain how I had kept depression at bay since I got the job at Excel. It just happened and I felt lucky that it hadn't returned. I was glad, but unsatisfied not understanding what happened. I wanted to dissect it, but I reminded myself again not to think too much about it. Was that it? Was that the key? I shook my head, feeling the tug to get lost in thought again.

I just had to focus on getting myself into a better position. That was an actionable thing and it made sense. If I was going to help them out, I still had debt to pay off and other projects to complete.

After Mom and Dad went home that Thanksgiving Holiday, I just focused on my work and doing a good job. I put my head down and got busy. If I wanted to make the kind of money I knew I would need, I had to bust my ass. I put my head down, worked, and had fun.

"Work Hard, Play Hard" became my motto. The little time I did have to play, I would usually be working on my car or out cruising in it. I hadn't touched ESO in months. I kinda missed my friends there, but I had wondered if not having time for video games was possibly a good thing, so I didn't really get back into it. Besides, with something like the RX-8 demanding so much of my time and attention, video games just paled in comparison.

Chapter 11

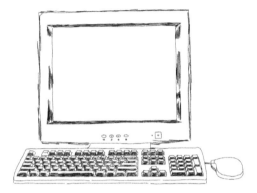

Two great years had gone by like this. Mom and Dad would bring Joseph down for Thanksgivings and Christmases, but Alex stopped coming with them. I did some stupid things in my car but had a blast doing it. Doing, and not thinking, seemed to be working?

I would experience sadness and other emotions, but those emotions seemed to be normal and made sense when they arose. It wasn't like before, where I just couldn't gain any emotional traction and the negative emotion would hang around for months. I was able to shrug things off and move forward with ease. I could rise to and meet my challenges with a confident understanding that I was doing my best. And that was enough. I wasn't worried about depression slipping back anymore because it had been gone for so long now.

But I had also gained something new: self-pride. When I first got the job, I accepted the position at $13/hr. I was just so happy and thankful to have the opportunity, that I didn't make a fuss about the money. In fact, I gave it very little thought to begin with. But after a couple of years, I got no raises and continued to work longer and longer hours in my salary position. I started to feel taken advantage of.

I decided to approach my boss about it one day, after weeks of nervously wondering whether I should say anything.

I knocked on Eli's office door, "Hey man. You busy?"

Eli looked up from his phone and pulled his legs off his desk, "Oh, hey Len. Nah, I'm not busy at all. What's up?"

I sat down in a chair in front of his desk, "So I was wondering how raises work here. I've been here for a couple of years now and I think I've done really well with the library contract and a couple of the other bigger contracts we have..."

Eli sat on the edge of his chair and interrupted me, "Oh man, no you're doing an amazing job. I have no complaints about your performance at all. Give me a few months to see what I can work up for a raise. Keep it up!"

That felt anti-climactic and weird... but he had no complaints and he asked me to give him a few months, so what was there to argue with? "Well... all right. I'll just keep doing what I do man."

Eli smiled, "Thanks, Len. Well, it's 4:30. You know what that means?" He put his hands, palm down, on his desk.

I chuckled, "Hah, yeah, time to go home." Inside, that made me lose so much respect for Eli. He would show up at 9AM and leave as early as 3PM some days. Meanwhile, we were working lots of extra hours trying to complete all the work. But I had to keep my attitude in check.

Eli nodded, then closed his laptop and pulled it off the dock, "Yep! Have a good night, Len. I'll see you tomorrow."

I marched out of Eli's office and went back down to the tech bench. We had one computer there that needed some work, then I could go home. It just needed all the data backed up, then a new hard drive and Windows installation. I started the data backup, put a new hard drive into the laptop, and got Windows installed. It was 5 minutes of work and about 3 hours of waiting, so I decided to head home. It wasn't 5PM yet, so I was technically getting out early for once.

Feeling good, both proud for having said something about my pay and getting out early, I practically skipped out to the car.

I sat down in the driver's seat and pulled out my phone, looking for Liz's number to call her and let her know that I was off work when I got an incoming call from Eli.

I excitedly answered the phone, naively hoping maybe he had already figured something out with the pay. "Hey man! What's up?"

Eli cleared his throat, "Hey man, listen. I just got a call from our local radio station. One of their new hires downloaded some sort of crypto-locking ransomware and it spread to the servers before anyone realized what was happening."

"Oh my god... no..." I lamented. I knew exactly where this was going.

"Yep." He assured me. "I need you to head out there and get on damage control. I'll be along to help in a little while."

I rubbed my forehead, "Yeah, sure. I'll get headed over there now."

Three hours later, Eli and Dale arrived. They brought me some cold McDonald's burgers, but that was better than nothing... debatably.

"Thanks." I said, looking down into a rather large McDonald's bag with two burgers in the bottom of it.

Eli clapped his hands, "So, where are you at? What's the situation?"

I inhaled and set the bag on a nearby desk with no intention of returning for it, "Every computer on this local network was infected, including servers. Damage control was a bust before I even got here. I've already got the servers restoring from our latest backups now. They're only going back a few days on their servers, but all the client machines need to be wiped and none of the employees have any backups of any of their stuff on those machines."

Eli looked at Dale and shook his head.

Dale turned around and waved, "Well, you boys have fun with that. I'm taking my old ass to bed where it belongs." And off he marched.

Eli looked back at me, "Alright. How many client PCs are we talking about here?"

"Seven." I was getting tired and hangry.

"Ok, ok..." Eli put his hand to his chin when his eyes suddenly lit up, "Ok, take all the client PCs to the office and put 'em on the tech bench. Reload them from the network image so you can do them all at once. If the employees didn't back up their data, there's nothing we can do now. It's crypto-locked, right?"

I shrugged, "Yeah, it's crypto-locked. Not sure how to get around that without a key."

Eli put one hand on each of their servers, "And these... just get Team Viewer installed on them and let the backups finish. I'll get Troy to connect to them in the morning and make sure they're configured properly." He nodded, looking satisfied with himself. "Ok, I'm out. See you tomorrow!"

I steamed as he ran off. I thought he was here to help me. Instead, he brings me three-hour-old barely-food, gives a couple of directions, and then immediately leaves. This selfish mother fu-

I realized I was staring at an empty hallway and being emotional when what I wanted to do was be done with this so I could go home. I shook my head and loaded all seven of the infected desktop computers up into my tiny RX-8.

I finally made it home around 10PM. I was trying not to focus on the fact that I did all that for free basically. Overtime was becoming more and more commonplace. Dale was selling services faster than we could perform them. From running cable to repairing computers and servers, we worked an average of about 60-70 hours per week. Anything over 40 each week was just free labor. Dale was getting bonuses off all his sales and really didn't care how many hours us salary employees had to work to get it all done. But we always did get it done.

Eli had developed a pattern. Every three months, I'd approach him and ask about the raise. Every three months, I'd get the same response. He'd just ask for a few more months to get it figured out.

"Hey... no, I have not forgotten." Eli defended himself.

I raised my eyebrow at him and cocked my head.

He put his hands up defensively, "I'm bringing options to my brother, he shoots them down, and I bring him more options. These things take time, man. I can't just give you a raise at the drop of a hat!" He was clearly defensive.

This might not go well if I keep pushing... "Whatever man." I said and walked out of his office. I had no respect for him anymore. I couldn't respect someone who thought they could lie to my face.

Starting to feel taken advantage of, my attitude started to get worse about working there. The other employees had issues with the pay and the hours too. We discussed it openly with each other and realized that he was doing each of us the same way. He'd tell each of us that he'd get it figured out in a few more months.

Out of us techs, Tyler had been there the longest. He let me know that's exactly how Eli had been doing him for the last 3 or 4 years now. There was no way I was about to play that game for that long. We knew Eli and Dale accepted handsome bonuses because they bragged about it to each other when they thought we weren't listening. It was no big secret in the office.

I needed to find another job, fast. So, I started looking around.

Over the course of a few weeks, I carefully looked around and hand-picked my best options. I interviewed, but never got any call-backs. I felt stuck. I could feel the depression coming back and my attitude at work was getting worse. This was no longer the good thing for me that it once was, but I exhausted all my choices.

I walked in the front door of the Excel office one day, looking at the ground as I walked. I was headed straight back to the tech bench and I wasn't going to really say much of anything to anyone. I was just going to do my job and go home.

Dale poked his head out of his office and hollered at me down the hallway, "Hey Len! Psst! C'mere!" He seemed jovial.

I set my things down at my cubicle in the tech room and went to Dale's office, "What's up man?"

He sat down and pulled himself up to his desk, "Have a seat. I've got some bad news."

I inhaled deeply and sat down at the empty chair in front of his desk. I simply made eye contact with him.

He played with one of his cufflinks, "This isn't an easy decision to make, but a lot of our bigger contracts have been completed and we need to lay 3 staff members off. You're the most established one, you'll be fine. The other folks here aren't as privileged as you are, so, we're letting you go first before we decide who the other two are. You don't need to report into work tomorrow, but we'll give you 3 weeks of pay while you look for something new. That's the least we can do. I'm really sorry. I wish we didn't ever have to have this conversation."

I felt pretty sure that story was 100% manufactured bullshit so we didn't have to address the real issue, my attitude because of the pay discrepancies. But I didn't care. I was suddenly overcome with happiness. I wanted out of that place so bad. I fought not to quit until I had something else lined up, and in this moment, I was just happy it was finally done, for better or worse.

I shook my head and stood up, "Oh man, no it's fine, really. I completely understand. Thank you for the few weeks of pay while I find something else." I kept it short and sweet, but equally as fake as the story he tried to sell me on. I just wanted out of the office as soon as possible.

Dale held up one hand, "Hold on, hold on... what about your jobs? Your contracts? Got any computers that need to be completed on the tech bench?"

I folded my arms, "You know my contracts. The Library, First Baptist Church, the Twins' clinic, Keith's place, and all the rest. And no, I don't have anything on the tech bench that's incomplete right now. I'll just go clear out my desk and hang around for about 45 minutes in case whoever is taking over my contracts has any questions before I'm gone." I wasn't going to train my replacement, but I'd give them a small window to get info from me before I left. I thought that was fair.

Dale reached out a single finger, "Ok, but wait. Please don't tell anyone you've been laid off. That includes employees and customers."

I shrugged, "Sure" and left his office.

I made sure I had all my things from the office collected in a box and then I sat at my now-empty cubicle for almost an hour browsing Reddit on my phone. I got up and tapped Dale's door, "Goodbye man. Thanks for everything." And I left. I didn't even wait for a response.

I was driving home at 2 PM. Liz wasn't even off work yet. I texted Liz and Jack that I'd gotten laid off before I left, but they were probably busy and hadn't seen the text yet.

I stopped at the liquor store on the way home and grabbed a bottle of Cannonball rum. I didn't even bother grabbing a shot glass. I just drank from the bottle. I was drinking partly in celebration, and partly in lament. The celebration was because I was out of that job and no longer had to be lied to. I hated it there. The lament was because I knew I was about to have to step up the job hunt and be ready to accept something maybe less than ideal at first and keep looking.

Liz and Jack both texted that they would head here ASAP, so I started drinking. I was already pretty drunk when they arrived.

Jack laughed as he walked into my office. "Well, hello." He waved.

I heard Liz say something, but I couldn't make it out because Moby was barking now. I was laying on the couch, on my back, and flipped my head upside down over the edge of the couch to see Jack standing in the doorway. "Oh hey maaaaaaaaan!" I said drunkenly.

The next thing I remember is waking up in bed the following morning around 9AM feeling like I'd been eaten and shat out by a T-Rex. I was miserable, but I was paying my stupid tax. I should not have drunk so much…

I decided I'd take that day for a recovery day and start job searching the next day. After many bottles of Gatorade and some chicken soup, I put out TONS of applications that week. I put applications out for positions I wasn't even qualified for just in case I got dumb-lucky with it. I put out applications I was way overqualified for, too. I was rapidly and unashamedly shotgun-blasting my resume across the town.

Seven days after I started searching, I got a call back from one of the jobs I had applied for.

I answered my phone, "Hello? This is Len."

"Hey, Len, this is Jordan, with Cyient. You may know my wife, Sabine. You worked with her at the Library."

I snapped with my fingers, "Oh yes! I know Sabine! She's awesome. I used her for a reference on this application."

Jordan started, "Yeah, so I saw your resume and talked to her about you. She had nothing but good things to say. So, I'm gonna set you up an interview with our General Manager, Francis later in the week. I don't know when it will be, but I'll reach back out in a day or two to let you know when it gets scheduled for."

I didn't understand their internal process for setting up interviews, but that sounded like a positive thing. "Okay, yeah that sounds great, Jordan! Thank you so much! I look forward to hearing back from you soon!"

We hung up and I immediately started texting Liz. Before I was even done typing the message out, Jordan called me back.

I answered the phone again, "Hello? This is Len."

"Hey Len. Jordan again. I just talked to Francis, and if you could be down here for an interview tomorrow at 2 PM, that would be perfect." He was right to business.

I smiled, "I can make it happen. Not a problem."

"Ok, good. Listen..." He paused for a brief moment, "Just be yourself. Don't overinflate your experience. Be real. We don't have any real dress code here, but that's because we all take it seriously and don't abuse it. You don't have to dress in a shirt and tie but at least look like you care."

That seemed perfectly reasonable, "Okay, yeah. Will do." I replied.

We got off the phone and I was so excited. I was worried I would somehow fall into another three to six months of depression before I got another job. I couldn't be happier to avoid all that nonsense and get right into the next thing. But I had one tiny problem... I had been smoking weed nonstop for the last 3 years. There was no way I would pass a drug test any time soon.

I immediately called Jack.

"Hey dude, what's up?" He answered his phone.

I started with an exhale, "I need your help dude. I have an interview scheduled for tomorrow, but I also need to be able to pass a piss test..."

He started laughing, "Oh man, this is gold. Are you asking me what I think you're asking me?"

I sheepishly joined in his laughter, "Hah... yeah, I need you to pee for me dude... That's where we're at." It was kind of funny. "Like, I'll go get... I dunno... I guess I'll get one of those water bladders for like a Camelback, but the cheap Walmart equivalent because this will not be re-used."

Jack kept laughing, "I mean, of course... you know I got you. But... it's just hilarious when you think about what's going down. This feels like a Seth Rogan movie all of a sudden."

I inhaled after I finally stopping laughing, "Thanks, dude. I owe you one. I'll be at your place around 10 AM tomorrow morning with a couple of energy drinks. Drink some water before I get there, and we'll pound the energy drinks together."

And so I did. I showed up around 10 AM with a small water bladder, some duct tape, and two Monsters. I knocked on his door and waited for him to come answer it.

He opened the door, stretching and yawning as he did so, "Morning man."

I raised my eyebrows and exaggerated my smile, "You ready to pee for me?" I held up the energy drinks and snickered.

He looked up and covered his face with his hand, "Oh my god, hahaha... yes, come on in man."

I stepped in, laughing. "Man, thank you for this, I really do mean it."

He walked back to his office and we talked and drank liquids for a couple hours until he really had to pee. He filled up the water bladder, sealed it, crimped the straw, and gave me the bag of pee. That stuff was glowing toxic green, I swear. My pee probably wasn't gonna look any better, but at least this stuff would pass a drug test.

Luckily, it was the middle of summer in the south, so the sun would keep the contents of the bag warm if I kept it on my dashboard. So, I did the interview and then got the papers to go take the drug test. The whole time during the interview, I just kept getting worried about the bag melting in the sun somehow and spilling its contents all across and into my dashboard. I tried not to let it distract me, but it was very hard.

After the interview, I ran out to my car to make sure no tragedy had occurred out there during the interview. I was safe. The bag was intact, and very warm... When I arrived at the clinic, I grabbed the bag of pee, and immediately dropped it back onto the dash. Did I mention it was warm? I meant it was hot. It was dangerously hot pee. I had to wait a few minutes for it to cool down before I could attach it to my leg with the duct tape.

This was risky... I had to make sure the paperclip didn't come off the hose, or it would leak pee. I made it through the drug test and took the stamped papers back to the Cyient office and finally back home, where I was finally able to untape this thing, painfully, from my thigh.

Chapter 12

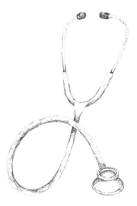

One week later, I got a call back from Francis.

I answered my phone, "Hey, this is Len."

Francis's voice came through the other end, "Hey Len! How's it going?"

"Hey Francis. I'm pretty good, I do believe." I answered confidently.

He laughed, "Good. Hey look, let's get you started. I'm looking at a passed drug test and a passed background check. I figure we'll start you at fifteen-fifty per hour if that sounds good to you. Then we do a yearly raise and I try to have my guys up to the pay-cap for their position within a couple of years. When do you want to start?"

Surprise overtook my face, "Wow... that sounds amazing. I'm sure I've got a lot to learn, but I'm not afraid of learning and working for it. Umm, let's get started first thing Monday if that works for you guys."

"That's perfect, Len." He said, "I'll see you then."

I hung up the phone and immediately started bubbling over with excitement. I couldn't believe I'd gotten so lucky. I was only out of work for two weeks before I was right back into an even better job.

Right from the start, Francis seemed like a leader worthy of my loyalty. I wore my fake plug earrings and just jeans and a T-shirt to the interview and it didn't matter at all to him. Jordan had told me to be myself, so I did, and I was pleasantly surprised to find a group of mature adults for once.

My first day on the job was awkward, as they always are. I introduced myself to 15 new people and forgot each of their names mere minutes after the introduction. The place seemed pretty laid back though. I had arrived at 8, and there were still people trickling in after me all the way up until 9 AM.

I was told to find and sit with Jerry, and that he would show me the ropes. So I walked around meeting people until I met Jerry.

I shook a man's hand who was wearing a grateful dead T-shirt, had long hair down his back, and had a thick beard that completely covered his neck from the front. "Hey Len, I'm Jerry."

My eyes lit up, "Aha! Hey Jerry, good to meet you. I've been told you're the man with the plan who's gonna teach me a thing or two?"

He laughed and shrugged, "I'm not the world's greatest teacher, but that's the idea. How much do you know about what we do? Got any experience in Telecom?" He waved me to follow him and turned to walk. "C'mon."

I started following, "No, unfortunately. I have a background in IT though, so I'm hoping that helps me pick it up quicker. Give me the rundown. What do we do?"

Jerry nodded slowly, "Ok, check it out. Right now, the government is giving big ISP's a bunch of money to develop high speed fiber connections to rural parts of the country. It's happening across all states and ISP's – you know what an ISP is right?"

I smiled and nodded my head, "Yeah, you're talking about an internet service provider, right?"

Jerry snapped his finger at me, "Exactly! Well, the ISP's come to us and say, 'We need your company to engineer roughly five-hundred-thousand feet of new fiber cable.' And give us a huge package of info. We call that the handoff package. And every handoff package should contain the same basic set of information." Jerry started fishing through his emails.

I popped one of my knuckles with the pen I was holding in my hand, "That makes sense. I'm guessing the handoff package has everything we need to follow contained in it?"

Still clicking around his inbox, Jerry tilted his head, "Yeah... that's the basic idea. The ISP will have a team of planners do a bunch of preliminary research and get approximate footages, but it's up to us to take that information to the field and measure everything out and plan through all the issues out in the field. We send someone out to get measurements. It's one guy in a van, but we've got a LiDAR machine strapped to the top of the van. So we just get our fielder to drive past the pole line or route we'll be placing the fiber, then we can review that data back here in the office and take exact measurements of all the field assets. He also takes pictures, so you can virtually drive the route kinda like the Google Maps Street View and see the field conditions for yourself as you engineer a job."

I was eating this up. This was so cool and nerdy. "Oh I see. So we send someone out to collect information from the field, then we take that data and design the job?"

Jerry triumphantly double-clicked the email he found. "Gotcha! Here, look at this. This is one of the handoff packages we got from Frontier for this job we're about to look at. Look at how general everything is. This tells us where we are starting from and where we are going to. But we have to make sure the path they have laid out will work. If it won't work, we have to work with them to figure out a solution and keep the job in budget still."

I scrunched my eyebrows with concern, "I'm not going to have to go to the field, am I?"

He looked at me and shook his head, "No, not at all. We have a guy who does that and he loves it. More power to him. I've got a kid on the way, so there's no way you're seeing me in the field any time soon. My wife would kill me." He laughed.

I nodded my head and snickered, "Okay good. I can't really be gone either. We don't want any wives doing any strangling in our sleep." I joked. "So where do I come in?"

A paper ball suddenly flew past Jerry's head and hit the computer monitor in front of us.

"He shoots, he scores!" A new voice rang out from across the room.

Jerry smiled and winked at me, then grabbed the paper ball and turned around, "Damn kids! All you do is play!" Without looking, he opened the drawer of his desk and dropped the paper ball into it. Then fished out... a...

nerf gun? He fired multiple nerf darts at the offending thrower of paper. "Take that!" He said, laughing heartily. He got up and walked over to the guy's desk, "Ok Blake, now gimme my darts back. Don't make me beat you for 'em!" He hadn't stopped laughing since he started firing the darts.

Jerry came back to the desk and had a silent "I see you" sign-language standoff with Blake before he turned to me laughing, "I promise we're adults and we actually make money around here." He joked, laughing and grinning.

Blake walked over to us and introduced himself, "Sup man, I'm Blake." He offered a handshake.

I shook his hand in return, "Hey Blake, I'm Len. Good to meet you."

Blake poked Jerry and pointed at me, "I'm gonna run down to the gas station real quick and grab a muffin and some orange juice. Either of y'all want anything?"

Jerry looked at his watch, "Damn son, you just got here!"

Blake looked at Jerry with a dead-pan expression, "Uh huh... and you know we'll be here until ten o'clock tonight, too."

Jerry made slapping motions at Blake, "Shhh, we're trying not to scare off our new hire! Hahahaha!"

I started laughing too, "No I'm good dude. Thanks for the offer though."

Blake shook his head and smirked, "Aight I'll be back." And he left.

I looked back at Jerry, "So nobody cares if we just run to the gas station or something real quick?"

Jerry shook his head, "Nah, not at all. As long as everything gets done at the end of the day, you can do what you gotta do. If you gotta get your oil changed, or you gotta go pick up your wife or something, it's all good. Just let someone know and make sure everything gets finished at the end of the day and nobody has any issues. We're pretty laid back here."

That sounded too good to be true. Everywhere else I worked, the leadership was paranoid and ultra-controlling of the worker's time. "Man, look, I just came out of a job where I was on salary, working 60-70 hours a week. As long as I'm getting paid for my time, I don't mind working long hours."

Jerry winced, "Careful brother. Don't let his place burn you out. That's why we have nerf guns and take breaks whenever we need them. This job can eat up a lot of your time if you let it. But anyway, you come in here..." He handed me a set of construction prints, "Look right here..." He pointed to some codes that were listed on the side of the page. "These are CAS codes. What they mean isn't very important right now, but what we need is just basic data entry. Someone will check this information to make sure it's accurate, then give it to you. Once you have it, we need you to enter all these codes and quantities into a piece of software called Infinium." He double-clicked several times on his computer and signed into two different pop-up windows, "This is the software you'll be using."

I watched his screen and took notes, asking TONS of questions. I understood that my job was to enter that data. But I wasn't personally satisfied with that being the end of it. I wanted to learn how this whole process worked, from start to finish. I was overcome with an insatiable curiosity.

I worked with Jerry this way for about a week, then I was on my own. I didn't get off work until Jerry did, so I put in nearly 80 hours my first week, and close to 100 hours the week after that. We were backed up with work for my position, so I could basically stay and work as long as I wanted. I still bugged Jerry with my questions, and he would teach me.

My first six months went by so fast... I worked 5 days a week, but I would be there from 6AM until 11 PM or Midnight sometimes. I was rarely alone as we all had a TON of work to complete. I got their entire backlog of data entry caught up and started to help with the design prints. I knew what all the codes meant already from entering them, so I just had to learn the civil engineering side of it. I knew how all the technology worked already, so that was just a matter of learning the right names and acronyms for things in this industry.

I had become comfortable in my role there and just focused on the work. I still had about $20k in debt that I needed to work off, and this overtime was getting me somewhere. All I had to do was keep it up.

I was at work one day and Alex called me, so I stepped outside to smoke a cigarette and talk with him.

I answered my phone as I exited the building, "Heyyyy bud!"

Alex sounded excited, "Hey Len! What're you up to?"

I opened my car door and sat down in my driver's seat, "Not much, bubba. Just taking a break at work and sitting down to talk with you. How you doin'? You sound excited."

He chuckled sheepishly, "Yeah, I'm doing better. I've got my own place now."

I nearly gasped, "No shit!" I was pleasantly surprised. "That's amazing news bud!"

"But wait," He continued, "It gets better. I'm living with my girlfriend and she's got a little girl! I'm kinda like a dad now. She's such a sweet little girl, too."

I didn't know how to respond, "Bud... wow... I can't believe it... How's the drug stuff coming?"

He chuckled again, "I haven't had any opioids or meths in 6 months."

Meths? I figured he was stealing prescription opioids from Mom, but he was doing meths, too? "Wow, that makes me incredibly happy to hear you've been off those. How'd you do it?" I was sort of confused. He went from struggling in most areas of his life to taking on a family and his own place within 6 months. I was proud, but also incredibly curious.

"I, uh..." He hesitated, "I had to go on a methadone program. I knew I needed to get a job, so I had to quit doing heroin, but you can't just quit heroin cold turkey."

Oh my god... Heroin? I almost panicked. "Damn bud, that's serious." I said without really thinking about it.

Alex continued, "Yeah but I got a job."

This conversation was pulling me all over the place emotionally. "A job? That's excellent! Where at? What do you do?"

He sounded proud, "I work at the hospital on the night shift. I'm a nurse's assistant. I do a lot of cleaning and delivering things, but I like it."

A wide smile spread across my face, "That's excellent! Damn bud, I didn't know things had gotten so bad up there, but I'm glad you're doing better. Man, wow..." I was both happy and worried at the same time. That was a lot of news about Alex that I just took in. I needed another cigarette already.

He sounded full of genuine concern, "I know you were worried about me, and you had good right to be, but I told you I was gonna be okay and I'm trying to be okay."

The wide smile stayed plastered across my face, "I'm so proud of you, bud. You're doing awesome. Just keep it up. That's all you gotta do now. Most of the hard choices are behind you and I'm excited for you. I'm so excited for you..."

I tried my best to make sure he knew how proud I was of him. I knew it took some hard choices, harder ones than I originally thought if he quit heroin, and I respected him for the strength I knew that took. We hung up, and I finished my third cigarette and walked back in.

Francis stopped me on my way past his office, "Hey Kester!" He hollered behind me, trying to get my attention.

I spun around, "Yo?"

He waved me back toward him with his hand, "Come here."

I nodded and started walking. "Aight, right behind ya." I said and followed him back to his office.

He shut the door behind me and went to his chair behind his desk, "Have a seat, "He waved at the chair in front of his desk as he passed it.

I sat down, "What's up man?" I said, overcome with curiosity. All the theatrics had me slightly nervous.

He pulled out his pen and started chewing on it between sentences, "You have done amazing. Couple of things. First, I'm bumping you up from fifteen-fifty per hour to seventeen-fifty per hour. You've certainly earned it. Second, do you know any more people like you who catch on quick and aren't afraid to work hard?" He started laughing.

I started laughing, too. The nervousness had vanished, and now I was just feeling embarrassed and unsure how to take the compliment, "Wow... uh... first of all, thank you for the raise. That means a lot to me. The last place I worked gave me the run around for a couple years." I thought, "And as for the second question, I do know of one person right now that I can highly recommend." I said confidently.

He leaned forward with his phone in his hands, "Who? Just tell me. I'll call 'em right now!" He started laughing.

"My little brother, Joseph." I said proudly. "He and I are both really into computers and he's incredibly smart and mature for his age. He's stuck in northern Indiana right now, and I'd love to bring him down here where there's at least a few more opportunities than where he is now."

He winced, "How old is he?"

I laughed, "He's 19 now, he's legal to work don't worry."

He looked relieved, "Oh good... I have to be legal here, Len!" He joked.

I surrendered my hands into the air, "Uh, sure, whatever you say, Boss Man." And broke into laughter again.

"When can he get down here for an interview?" He asked.

I made a funny face, "Well... he's in Indiana at the moment. We'll be moving him down here for this if he gets it. I can go ahead and move him down, then we can do the interview and drug test."

"Do you have all the other details figured out?" He asked, still chewing on his pen.

"Yeah," I nodded, "He can stay with me and I can bring him into the office with me until he gets his own place and car. He can take as long as he wants on that. Let me call him tonight and ask him what he thinks."

Francis pulled the pen out of his mouth, "Okay, great. Let me know what he says. Oh, by the way, I almost forgot, I'll be giving you your own crew and projects now, too."

I nearly choked, "W- M... Me?"

He nearly doubled over laughing so hard, "Yeah. We need you to start on the next Frontier contract. But all the guys that were on the team with you last time have to go to the AT&T team for a new contract over there. I need you to train a few new guys to do what JR and his guys did with you."

I exhaled sharply, "I need to get out of your office before I end up with more responsibilities!" I joked.

When I got out of work that night, I was flooded with good emotions. Alex was doing well, and I had a legitimate opportunity to move Joseph down to Mississippi with me and right into a good job. So many things were going right. I could only be thankful.

That night after dinner, I called Joseph.

"Hey bud, what'cha up to?" I asked after he answered his phone.

He sighed, "Oh, nothing really. Just playing some video games with Kohl. What're you up to?"

"Well, uh..." I paused, wondering if I should just throw it all at him or ease in with some small talk. I decided to just lay it out there and save the small talk for when it was needed. "I'm good, really good in fact, but how would you like to move down here to Mississippi and get a job with me as a Telcom Engineer? You'd be starting at almost seventeen an hour. You could stay at my house, rent free, as long as you like. We'll move the computers out of the office and into the living room, and you can have the office for your bedroom. Save up your money, buy a car, get your own place, whatever you wanna do. What do you think?"

Silence hung in the air for a moment as he thought, "How long do I have to decide?"

That was a good question... I hadn't thought about it before now. "I don't have an exact answer for that question, but I'm sure you've got a couple weeks. You have time to think about it if you need the time."

"Phew, okay, because I was just sitting here playing video games and wasn't expecting all that, haha." He started laughing.

I shook my head and laughed too, "I'm sorry, I didn't mean to catch you off-guard like that. I just don't see a point in holding something like that back for small talk. Take all the time you need bubba."

We got off the phone and I kept my fingers crossed for the next few days.

Chapter 13

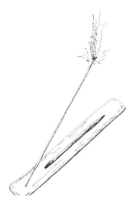

I came home and set my keys on the counter, "Phew!" I exhaled. "Another year's fiber builds done! We completed one point-two million feet of fiber placement, the team and me." I shook my head in disbelief.

Liz balked, "Wow, that's... quite a bit. Well, you have spent a lot of time at work... so... it does make a certain amount of sense."

Joseph spun around in his computer chair, "Wait, one point-two... MILLION..."

I walked into the front room, where all of our computers had been moved to after Joseph moved in, and sat down at my computer, pulled out my jar of weed, and rolled a joint. "Yup... One point-two-friggin'-million feet!" I did a soft fist pump. "I'm gonna have Dipak, Siddhartha, and Chandra over for a barbecue. You know they told me today they've never had an American invite them over to their house for dinner?" I shook my head.

"Oh shit... really?" Joseph drooped his head and hunched his shoulders slightly, "That's kinda sad."

"Yeah..." I licked the rolling paper, "So I'm gonna fix that. We showin' them what Kester BBQ is all about!" I cackled. "Uh, Joseph, when do you go out of town again?" Joseph could be out of town for weeks at a time, so I loved it when he was home.

"Uhhh…" He had to think, "We've got to head to Birmingham on Monday, so I've got all weekend to be here at home."

"Nice!" I fist-pumped again and put the joint in my mouth, "Kester Thanksgiving 2016 is just around the corner, too! I'm excited." I was always hyper and sort of manic when I came home from work. Smoking weed didn't necessarily help that, but smoking it was still something I did anyway. It simply took time to calm down and just be at home for me to relax and get hungry, so I'd smoke a joint and take a few minutes to relax on the front patio. I didn't like smoking anything inside because it left a nasty, sticky residue on the walls.

Nobody wanted to join me, so I went out to the patio alone. I was okay with being alone sometimes. It gave me time to think and reflect, which I had decided a little bit of was ok. I sat out on the patio and I thought about the next couple of car upgrades I wanted to do to the RX-8, then my thoughts rolled back around to Alex. I hoped like hell he was still doing good. It was already late, but I sent him a text anyway.

"Love you bud! Hope you're doing good!" I'd hoped that would brighten his day a little bit, even if he didn't reply.

Even after smoking and relaxing, I still wasn't hungry, so I just decided to head for bed.

Something felt whole or complete when Liz and Joseph and Moby were all around me. I wished Alex and Donny were there, too. It would only make me feel more whole and complete. Someday, I wanted to be able to afford to build a series of houses on some land somewhere in the woods where we could all live together. It was a silly dream, I knew it, but it made me happy to think about.

The months went by quickly. I stayed busy, and Joseph stayed gone 80% of the time. I missed him most of the time, but it was good for him to travel while he was young and had no attachments. Another government-funded year of fiber builds was underway, and we had grown as a team. We had other markets that had grown as well, so we had moved to a bigger building.

In this new building, the 5 managers had individual offices. The rest of us had to be in what we all called "the fishbowl". The fishbowl was a large, open room with about 40 desks in it. When one person was on a phone call, everything going on in the background could be heard. It was a mess.

Francis was pacing around the office with another manager named Chris. They would do this when there was a problem that needed an immediate solution. Francis would pace around, and Chris would follow him.

Francis paced past my desk, "Yeah, that would work, but then we would still need someone to drive up to Ohio and run that second LiDAR van so we can keep collecting field data in that region. Who the hell is just going to want to operate an MX2 that you would also trust to operate it?" He looked at Chris.

Dipak and I both looked at each other and started laughing. We both motioned to each other to raise our hands and volunteer to go. We weren't serious, but we thought it would be funny because we were basically saying the office sucked so much that we'd rather be out in the field away from our friends and family. There was no way he'd let either of us out of the office. Another hour, another harmless joke.

Dipak and I both flailed our arms in the air like 9-year-olds volunteering during gym class. "Oh, pick me, pick me, pick me!" We said together, but not in unison. We stopped and started cackling like schoolgirls once we knew they saw us.

Francis came over to our desks and Chris followed, "You guys are nuts. I have a hard enough time letting you out of the office so you can go home, let alone to Ohio for 2 weeks." He spun on his heel and raised a hand to wave us off but paused mid-stride. "Wait..."

Dipak and I looked at each other. "Uh oh..." I said.

"This is not good, Len..." Dipak said, fighting laughter.

Francis spun back around to face us, "Len, you have an IT background... You also pick up on new things quickly... Dipak knows his shit, right?" He looked serious.

Feeling put on the spot, I responded obviously, "Well, of course. Dipak's the man." I looked over at Dipak who had just stood up, and he was looking at Francis with dejection. Then I realized in horror that yes, I said something good about Dipak, but I also just inadvertently threw him under the oncoming bus I didn't see until this moment. Dipak looked at me long enough to cast a little bit of sadness before shaking his head and sitting back down.

"Oh no..." I panicked internally, "Dipak can't do this alone. I wouldn't be able to do it alone, either. I need Dipak's help, and he needs mine. We work as a team." I changed my tone to sound sly and playful, "That's how we work miracles, right Dipak?" I looked over to Dipak for some support.

"Hah! No, no, no..." Francis laughed and waggled his finger, "Good try. It'll just be for a couple of weeks. That's it...."

Six months later, I was desperate to get out of the field and back home to Liz. Seeing her once or twice a month was starting to trigger my depression again. I couldn't have that on the road. I couldn't have that anywhere, but the road was among the worst locations to have the depression strike.

I was driving slowly because we were driving on a dirt road through a Blizzard in a white, one-wheel-drive, Ford Transit Van.

"Ohhh myyyyy goooood..." I worried out loud as the snow piled higher and higher and visibility grew less and less.

Jack gripped the support handle above the passenger's window, "Just don't stop. We can't afford to lose momentum right now..."

I leaned forward in my seat, fully alert, "I'm not planning on stopping. I just hope nothing stops me for me. I don't have a whole lot of traction or visibility right now." I could feel the single rear wheel slipping and transferring power between the two sides.

"Naw, we're fine." He assured me, "Just don't stop..."

I never stopped and about 35 minutes later, we made it back out to a main road, and another 40 minutes had us back on the Interstate. We had left out of Bar Harbor, Maine, and were headed for Logansport, IN. That's nearly a 20-hour drive, so we got up at 4 AM and started the trip early.

"I can't believe we got out of that snowstorm in one piece in this one-wheel-drive van." Jack started laughing.

I gripped the steering wheel, "Man, that was wild. You couldn't force a greased marble up my ass while we were driving through that nonsense. 100 different things could have gone wrong, and we'd still be out there stuck in it." I shuddered, "But I'm glad we made it out alright. We're even on time still." I was excited to see Mom, Dad, and Alex in Logansport, but I really missed Liz and couldn't wait to be home ultimately.

I sighed, "Jack, dude, I gotta be honest man. I love you and being out in the field with you these past 6 months has been awesome. We've seen some fun moments, and we've seen some moments that took a lot to get through. I wouldn't trade the experience for anything, but I need to be off the road for a couple of weeks. I think I'm gonna talk to Francis and ask him if I can have the time off, but most likely I'll have to work in the office for a couple weeks to make it work."

Jack reclined his seat and put his boot on the dash, "Man... you know if you go back into the office you're never coming back out to the field, right?"

I cocked my head. I hadn't considered that, but I was desperate for a break. "Man, I don't want to abandon you, but I need some time to spend with Liz. I'm not cut out for life on the road. I at least need a couple weeks every so often... I mean... I committed my life to that woman, not just three to five days a month, y'know?" I was feeling defensive because I felt guilty. I knew there was a chance I could never return to the field if I went back into the office, and that would leave Jack alone out in the field, unless he looked for another job. I didn't want to put that on him, but I was also headed for a bad place if I stayed out on the road for weeks at a time with just a couple days off to wash clothes and see my wife every few weeks.

Jack dropped his head and nodded, "I hear you; I'm just saying... You got me on here specifically so we could travel together. If he keeps you off the road, then this is just gonna suck for me."

I felt terrible. I felt like Jack was going to think I was just being weak. The emotions that I could feel bubbling their way, uncontrolled, to the surface more and more often scared me. I hadn't ever figured out what I did to make the depression go away so long ago now, I was still terrified of it coming back. Caught between trying to do what's best for me and also what's best for Jack, I felt nothing but dread.

Then an idea hit me, "Oh dude, what if we get you moved into the office, too? Then you'd get to be home more often and wouldn't be stuck on the road?"

Jack shrugged, "I don't know if I'd get as much overtime in the office. And I doubt they'd give me a raise to come into the office. I don't know if I could make that work financially."

I pined. Was there really only one solution here that would work? I felt trapped, like if I chose to take some time off the road, I'd be turning my back on my friend in the worst way. I wasn't going to be any good to anyone if I fell into another depression slump either though. Plus, I knew Liz was missing me, too. What about her?

Damned if you do, damned if you don't.

On our first gas stop, Jack found this HUGE unicorn stuffed animal. It had to have been five feet in length from nose to tail. It was white, pink, and purple. He bought it for Tiffany, and the whole way to Mom and Dad's house, he would periodically recline his chair and puppeteer the giant unicorn to look and wave at cars and trucks as we passed them. It was hilarious. Any kids we passed loved it. One trucker honked at us a few times and I could see him laughing in his cab.

We got to Mom and Dad's house at around midnight. Mom and Dad were asleep, but Alex was awake and he helped us carry our stuff up.

Alex set my luggage down in the living room, "Anything else down there?"

I shook my head, "Nah, that's all of it." I hugged Alex, "Bud, what're you doing here? I thought you were living with your girlfriend and her daughter?"

Alex rested his head on my shoulder, "We broke up a few weeks ago. It's all good though."

I kept hugging him, "Aw bud. How you doin' about it? You okay?"

He shrugged in my embrace, "I mean yeah... I'll be fine. I got a job at Walmart working in one of the local distribution centers. I'm making good money, and I still have the Durango."

I released my hug, "That's good to hear. You still going to the methadone clinic?"

"Yeah," He nodded, "But it's really expensive. It takes almost my whole paycheck."

"Do you think the methadone clinic is necessary?" I asked curiously.

"Oh... oh, yeah... ohhhh yeah. If I don't stay on methadone, I'll go back to heroin and OD." He answered very quickly and defensively.

I raised my eyebrows in shock, "Wow... well, we definitely want to avoid heroin and OD'ing." I thought that his response just now felt an awful lot like conditioning. Like, if I were a methadone clinic that depended on that continued income, that's what I'd tell my patients, too. But I also knew that heroin and methadone were serious chemicals and you had to be smart about managing recovery. I didn't know what to think, but I knew that I didn't fully trust the methadone clinic to have Alex's best interest at heart.

"Oh, let me go clean up my room. Don't come in until I get it cleaned but give me a few. Then we can hang out and talk in there." Alex said excitedly.

I shrugged, "You know I don't care about your room being a little messy bubba. It's fine." I started to follow him.

He turned around and put his hands on my chest, stopping me, "No... just please trust me, let me go clean up my room. It might take me a minute."

I froze for a second, confused. "I mean, if it means that much to you... ok. I guess I can get my bed set up while you clean..."

"Thank you, Len. I'm sorry. I don't mean to be weird, it's just... it's a mess and I know how clean you are." He disappeared behind the curtain hanging in one of the adjoining doorways.

I looked at Jack with a confused look, "I dunno what that was about..."

Jack and I got settled in and started watching some TV on the couch. We were both exhausted, but I was trying to stay up, waiting for Alex to finish cleaning his room. It took him hours to get his room clean, but he finally did.

Alex flipped the curtains back and opened his door, "Hey Len, I'm ready."

I inhaled sharply, fighting the sleepies, "Oh okay, I'm coming." I stretched as I got up. I noticed Jack was already asleep beside me, so I didn't wake him up.

As I entered the room, it smelled amazing in there. Alex had lit some Nag Champa incense because he knew it was my favorite. I sat on his bed next to him and leaned my head on his shoulder, "How you doin', bubba?"

Alex shrugged uncomfortably, "I'm good. I promise. Sure, life is hard, but you know that. Have you heard of Joe Rogan?" He was quick to change the subject.

I struggled with wanting to press further into his personal life, "Yeah, I've heard of Joe Rogan. The comedian, right? Didn't he start a podcast recently or something?"

Alex nodded excitedly, "Yeah, but like... he's just a dude. His podcast is cool because he doesn't have anyone telling him what he can or can't talk about, so he just talks about anything. Here, look at this one he does with Alex Jones. There's some crazy shit in here dude..."

I was happy to see Alex excited, but I was also disappointed. I wanted to talk about him. I wanted to know how my little brother was doing underneath all the struggles, but he just wanted to talk about Joe Rogan's podcast and all the crazy conspiracy theories he found there. I decided to just be glad for the moment, but I was also exhausted. We talked about Joe Rogan's podcast for about another hour and a half before I had to pass out.

"Good morning, Dad!" I squinted and smiled on my way into the kitchen to get coffee.

There was Dad sitting at the head of the table, as usual. He had an array of knives sprawled out in front of him and he was sharpening and oiling them. "Good morning, Big Guy! Did you sleep alright?" Dad put his knives and cloths down, then stood and walked into the kitchen with me. "That coffee is fresh by the way." He added.

That was music to my ears, "You're amazing." I hugged him when he met me, "Yeah, I slept alright. I was up pretty late talking with Alex, but once I hit the pillow, I was out. What's on the agenda for the day? I don't have to leave until tomorrow morning." I proceeded to pour a cup of sweet, sweet coffee.

He took his reading glasses off, "Well, we're gonna run into town and see the butcher. I'm gonna pick us up some steaks and we grillin', boy!" Dad's voice crescendoed with culinary delight.

Grilling was Dad's religion. It was the family secret that he tried to pass down to us. He could take a slice of chuck roast and make it taste like a New York Strip Steak somehow. From brisket to ribs, there was nothing he couldn't perfectly make every time.

Grocery shopping was an all-day thing, too. Jack and I went with Dad, and by the time we got back, we were so ready to start eating. Spending all day with Dad while he talked about the delicious meal that he's about to make had a way of getting to your stomach.

Jack clinked his fork down on his plate with the last bit of energy he could muster, "I need to go into a steak coma now so I can digest all that..." He started chuckling, "I'm so full..."

Dad nodded emphatically, "Yeahhhh buddy! Can't go wrong with steak, man. Can't go wrong with steak." He crossed his legs and lit a cigarette, beer in-hand. Dad was the only person I know who could have a lit cigarette and an open beer in his hands at all times and still be 100% functional.

I finished my last bite of steak and looked at Dad, "Hey, if I quit smoking...

would you quit too?" I smiled and hoped it didn't sour the air too much. Dad didn't like people giving him shit for things he enjoyed doing.

Dad slowly shook his head, "Buddy, I might quit one day. But not today."

I laughed and nodded, "Fair enough. I figured it was worth the effort to try." I lit a cigarette of my own. "Jack and I need to get headed out pretty early, so we'll be heading to bed real soon. If I don't see you in the morning, I love you, Dad."

Jack and I got our clothes folded since we were able to do laundry while we were there and got as much packed into the van as we could before bed.

The morning came early. Jack and I drove back home. He and I made probably 6 or 7 visits out to Mom and Dad's house while we were driving all around that part of the country. Every time we came up here, it was the same experience. Dad was excited to see us and would roll out the red carpet. Alex would spend a few hours cleaning his room. And Mom would be asleep almost the entire time.

I deeply admired Dad for his ability to do something he said he would, no matter how hard it got. He kept his commitments, he didn't complain, and he always went above and beyond for his family. He taught me by example to 'embrace the suck' as they say in the military.

Chapter 14

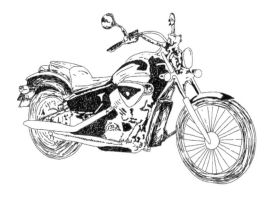

I stood in Francis's Office, frustration welling up inside, "No, Francis, it's not a permanent thing. I don't mind being out on the road, but, man, I need time at home. I'm glad I can be useful out there, and all the windshield time is easy money, but I married that woman for a reason. I happen to really like spending my time with her at the house that we purchased together." I attempted to reason.

"Oh my god…" Francis's words were hurried and frustrated, "I can't afford to just pull the van out of commission whenever you feel like being home." He protested.

I shook my head, "This was supposed to be temporary anyway. I didn't get hired on as a LiDAR operator or field agent, but I'm doing the best I can with the options I'm being given here. And you don't even want to get me started on the pay issues again." I warned.

He put his hands up, "Yeah, I know, I'm still trying to fix the pay issues. But I need things to function still while I chase that stuff down." His voice sounded desperate and frustrated.

I nodded, "And I have done my best for 6 months man. This was not supposed to carry on this long in the first place. Getting to see Liz for 4 or

5 days a month is not at all what I had in mind when I married her." I was desperate and frustrated, too.

He waved his hand at me, "And it was gonna be temporary until you got Jack hired on as your partner."

"Was that a hidden ultimatum you didn't tell me about?" I accused him angrily, "I asked you to hire someone I trusted because it was clear to me that you weren't going to let me back off the road like you said you were." I was growing more frustrated. "And instead of backing off and letting me stay in the office, you hired someone new just to keep me on the road. You know I haven't ever stopped helping Dipak run the show? I'm still on all the conference calls, I'm still writing scathing emails to Offshore at night, and I'm still figuring everything out with Dipak. My workdays are no less than 12 hours, but usually 16." I realized I was angrily rambling, so I exhaled in frustration.

Francis balked at me, "Oh whatever, you don't work that many hours."

"Excuse me?" I blinked. "You don't check the time entries, do you?"

He laughed and shrugged, "I usually bulk approve because I don't have time to check them all."

I nodded, "Uh huh... Well, I've never lied to you and I'm not about to start now. I'm gonna burn out man. I need some time. I know you're used to someone being out on the road permanently and alone, but I'm not that permanent answer." I was desperate for him to take me seriously.

"Yeah, ok. I'll let you have a couple weeks." He said nonchalantly. I could tell he wasn't happy with the direction the conversation was going.

I did a double take, "What? Just like that?" I wasn't necessarily complaining, but it felt off. "Was it something I said?" I knew I was pressing my advantage here, but I was emotional and being sarcastic. I knew there was a catch he wasn't telling me about, just like before when he hired Jack.

The catch ended up being that I was, in fact, never going back out on the road with Jack. As the next few months passed, I worked hard to get Jack off the road since I felt responsible for him being out there. But... things only got worse from there.

I looked up from my desk. I had gotten a rare hour to put my headphones in and focus on my personal to-do list. I folded my arms behind my head and stretched in my desk chair. Out of the corner of my eye, I noticed Chris was over at Jack's desk. My headphones were still in, so I couldn't hear what was being said. My team knew that if I had my headphones in, I was trying to focus on something that most likely had a deadline, and they would leave me alone to focus. But as soon as I took my headphones off, I would get swarmed with problems and questions that had been building up while I was working.

I wasn't ready for that tsunami of questions yet, so I left my headphones in and watched. Chris's body language looked irritated and accusatory. Chris threw his hands in the air and shook his head. While speaking, he was red-faced, so I could tell he was raising his voice to be heard across the fishbowl.

This wasn't the first time Chris did this, in fact, he often put his least favorite employees on public blast in that room. I usually just ignored him because that's why Chris did it – he wanted an audience to look smart or cool to. But he was doing it to Jack now. This was one of my best friends. I wanted to break Chris's knees while I watched him treat Jack, a veteran Marine, like a child. The worst part of it was that I knew Chris was just using Jack to make himself feel better because of how sad and insecure this man was.

After a few minutes of arbitrarily berating Jack, Chris circled the fishbowl like a shark. He started walking over to my corner of the large room.

I had a female member of my team who had recently been transferred under me from Chris's team. She was young, attractive, and smart. She sat near me with the rest of the team members so I could run to their desks quickly and look at problems as they ran into them.

"Hey Samantha." Chris put one leg up on her desk and did the Captain Morgan pose. He put his crotch at eye-level with her and started talking, "You did a good job with that email, but I think I would have worded it just a little differently." He continued to pull pure opinion out of his ass and assert it like fact. I wondered if he realized how incredibly obvious it looked to the rest of us.

I pulled out one headphone, turned my chair to face them, and stared relentlessly at Chris. I knew he was trying to ignore me when we made the briefest eye contact for a moment. I continued to stare as uncomfortably as I could. What I was witnessing was not only pathetic, but unproductive. Chris was a married man, so I had even less respect for this behavior from him.

I knew that my staring would prevent him from really pushing anything, and eventually he went away. I made eye contact with Samantha after he left, and she just looked at me with confusion and shrugged. I inhaled deeply, trying to control my emotions. The right thing to do was to go to Francis, but what I wanted to do was to introduce a blunt object to Chris's kneecaps. I knew that If I started a fight with Chris, Jack would back me up in a heartbeat.

I couldn't start a fight though. I needed to think about my career. I marched into Francis's office after Chris went outside for a cigarette break. "Dude, this is fucking ridiculous. Chris runs around the office bullying anyone he feels like bullying. This is not okay." I was still pretty hot.

"Hey!" Francis instantly hit the ceiling, probably because I came in so hot. "You don't barge into my office and start talking shit about my leadership!"

I put my hands up and took a breath, "Fair enough, I did kinda barge in here in a fit. Let me back up and punt." I took another deep breath, "Dude, I respect you, but I just watched Chris berate Jack and give Samantha the "Captain Morgan" treatment again. You got him to quit snapping at us like dogs to get our attention, can you do anything about this behavior?" I snapped my fingers to mimic Chris's behavior.

Francis shook his head, "Jack is fucking up and Chris is putting him in his place. I've never seen him do that to Samantha, so I don't know what you're talking about."

I marveled. Was he really trying to just minimize everything and pretend it didn't exist? Was that his idea of managing? I shook my head, "Look man, I'm watching this stuff happen in front of me and it's not cool. It's just not okay behavior from someone who is supposed to be a leader."

Francis stood up and the veins in his neck and forehead became visible under his red skin, "I'm not here to manage your personality conflicts with my managers! You either get over it or don't, but he's here to stay!"

I found myself marveling again at a complete loss for words. Was he really refusing to see Chris's behavior? Did he think that if he just didn't see it or acknowledge it that he could then distance himself from it? Or did he really not believe it? He had a potential lawsuit on his hands with Chris, but he seemed to not care. I suddenly felt insecure working there for Francis. Throwing caution to the wind was our mantra, but this made me realize how deep that philosophy went.

Feeling minimized, I broke the silence, "Okay, what about my pay issues?" I reminded him, "My pay wasn't right before, and now, after this latest supposed fix, I'm thirty cents lower. Do you remember me telling you about that last week?"

Francis cocked his head in confusion, "You weren't joking?"

I put my head into my hands and started rubbing my forehead, "It's really frustrating that you never take me seriously and constantly minimize my concerns. No, I wasn't joking, man! My pay is even more fucked now, and yet my responsibilities keep going up. If I refused to perform my duties, there'd be hell to pay. But if the company refuses to compensate me, I'm just supposed to be okay with it? No, no, if the company takes me down in pay, I should be outright thankful? I still have the same title I got hired in as, yet I'm doing manager duties. How does any of that make any damn sense? What am I busting my ass for again?"

Francis shook his head, "No Len, it takes time. This isn't just some get-rich-quick-button you can smash for money."

My spine crawled. "What've I been doing for the last 4 years, Francis? Playing tiddly-winks for 16 hours a day 7 days a week? No, I've been busting my ass. And because we all bust our ass out there," I pointed out at the fishbowl, "you were able to announce last month that we've crossed 60 million in revenue last year. Is wanting a piece of that pie asking for a handout to you?" I was legitimately surprised, and frankly pissed.

Francis balked at me, "You think that's just 60 million that I get to put in my pocket? We have to pay bills, Len. That money goes back out as fast as it comes in."

I noticed a pattern in Francis's reactions that I wasn't impressed with. I exhaled sharply, "Here's some math that doesn't add up to me. We paid our bills and afforded regular raises for twenty-five employees when we made under one million. That was when I first got here. We have about a hundred and ten employees now. If we functioned well with the twenty-five employees making just under one million per year, then we should be able support that same structure at a hundred employees with a yearly gross income of 4, or even 5 million per year. Hell, ten million per year should give us lots of breathing room beyond what we had. We're making sixty million, Francis. That's nearly five-hundred thousand per employee. Why are we not seeing any of that revenue we were instrumental in generating? Where the hell is it going? It's going somewhere and it stinks."

Francis put his hands up, "Hey, it's not going to my pocket. I don't know what the company does with the money we make for them."

"I believe you dude," I put my pointer finger straight into the air, "But my point still remains. We're busting our asses and handing the majority of our lives over to this company and we're fighting for scraps. What happened man? When I first got here, I had a $2 raise within the first 6 months. That earned you my loyalty. Not Cyient. You, specifically. You did me right and I haven't forgotten that. But what happened?" I pined for reason.

Francis sighed in defeat, "Gah... look, I'll be honest. This place is getting rough. I keep talking to my bosses about the pay issues and they keep blowing me off. You're not the only one with pay issues. Once we increased our revenue by 10 times in one year, the big wigs swooped in and took all the control from me. I don't have exactly the same position I did then, but that's not your problem, so I can't really use that as an excuse can I?"

Finally, it felt like I was having a conversation with the guy I had come to know as a friend, and not my boss. It was an awkward relationship at times. "It's okay dude. All I expect from you is to just be honest with me and not hide the truth. That makes sense that the big wigs would want to get their fingers in the pie once they see how much we're growing. And I dunno, I guess that's their prerogative and all, but it's not exactly making me want to stay here and keep busting my ass for nothing." I slouched in my seat and exhaled.

Francis shook his head, "I'll make it right, Len. I will."

I appreciated his energy, but I really wished he wouldn't promise me things that we both knew were outside of his control.

Chris never treated Jack any better. Any time I approached Francis about it, my concerns were immediately minimized and I was turned back around. Jack eventually found another job a couple months down the line. I don't know what any self-respecting person would have done differently. Chris had worked hard to guarantee that Cyient was not a sustainable solution for Jack, for whatever reason.

Months later, I had to sell the RX-8 because it was just too expensive to maintain properly. I sold it and bought myself a Honda Shadow 650 Cruiser bike and got Liz a Nissan Juke, Black Pearl Edition. Since we lived in the hot south, I could just bundle up for the couple of months that it was cold and I'd be fine. With water resistant gear and waterproof coat, rain wasn't a problem either. I just needed to respect the physics of traction.

Feeling good about my still-new bike, I headed home and prepared to party a few weeks after Jack had gotten another job. It was a Friday and I had started organizing hangouts at my house on the weekends that I wasn't working through. It was really nice to unwind after a long week or two and get drunk with a house full of my friends. Work hard, play hard.

After everyone left the party, Jack stayed with me while I cleaned.

"... and so this cop passes us that way as me and this dude were racing this way and flips on his lights. But it's the interstate, so it's divided. The cop can't just whip around, he's got to go down to the next exit and turn around. So I punch it!" Jack started giggling, "I swear to God the car was trying to take off at one-thirty. I couldn't believe that big, wide-ass Challenger felt so weightless... it was kinda scary."

I scraped a mound of steak scraps off a plate and into Moby's food bowl, "Dude, that sounds wild. One time, when I was working at Excel, I got sideways through the Main Street and Gloster intersection in town in the RX-8." I put the plate into the sink and started to wipe down the counters.

"I don't even know who that other guy was, but he was in one of those new Hyundai Velosters. Those things can move." Jack grabbed a couple of fresh glasses and looked quizzically at me, "Wanna smoke the pipes and sip on some bourbon?" He asked.

I looked at the dirty counter and the sink full of dishes. Then I looked at the bottle of whiskey. I was already drunk, and I really didn't feel like cleaning right now... but it would bother me knowing it was a mess.... I shrugged, "Eh, fuck it." I said with a slight slur.

I sat down at the front patio table and swung an empty chair in front of me to post my legs on. I kicked back, and lit my pipe, "Mmmmm, spiced rum tobacco... I forget how good this is every time." I put the match in the ash tray and puffed. "So how's Waste Management treating you dude?"

Jack set his bourbon glass down, "Damn, that's good bourbon... uh, it's good man. It's actually pretty awesome. They like give me a task and leave me alone to complete it. If I have questions, I don't get treated like an idiot. I get trained. It's amazing how well that works, Hah!" Jack trailed off in laughter.

"Man, that's really good to hear. I'm so glad you got out of Cyient. I might need to do something similar soon." I sipped my bourbon.

Jack popped a single eyebrow, "Lookin' to get away man? I can't really say I blame you. There's better out there."

I swirled my bourbon idly, "Yeah, I thought this was gonna be the place I retired from. Things looked so promising at the start of the job." I took a sip and let my thoughts wander for a second, "Well, on second thought, the devil you know, right? Maybe it's best to just stay here after all. I mean, think about it. I'm established here, and yeah, they'll keep jerking me around about the pay, but where the hell else am I gonna go? I don't want to change careers again. I could do it if I had to, but it takes a lot of energy to front load all the learning just to get taken advantage of in the end anyway." I leaned my head back against the chair.

"Man, I know they didn't treat you as bad as they treated me, but they still do you wrong." Jack looked at me through the candlelight, shadows dancing across his face.

I shrugged and lifted my head from the chair, "Well, yeah, they treat me wrong. I'm a cog in a machine. Isn't that the same no matter which company I go work for? I'm beginning to think a 'benevolent businessman' is rarer than bigfoot or Atlantis. I mean, I see Francis's predicament. He's a cog in a machine too, right? So what do you do? You stick with what you know. Besides, I'm pretty invested in the relationship I've built with the folks up at Frontier in Ohio. I haven't done everything flawlessly, but I've spent so many hours caring for that account and those customers. It's... it's like my baby. I dunno... I guess I'm not ready to throw in the towel on it yet."

He stroked his beard, "I get that, I get that. If you do ever want to get away from Cyient, just let me know. I got you man."

"Thanks man," I raised my glass to him and took another sip, "I love you man. I really appreciate you." I suddenly became aware that I had reached 'that' level of drunk, but I pressed on anyway. "Thanksgiving is coming up again in a couple weeks. Mom and dad are coming down and they're bringing Alex with them this time! Alex hasn't been down in a few years, so it'll be nice for all of us to be together again. I'd love for you, Tiffany and Logan to be there, too man."

Jack bobbed his head up and down, "Oh niiice man. Yeah, I'll be there. Is your Dad smoking a turkey again this year?" He finished the last of his bourbon.

"Ohhh yeah," I drew the words out, "We can't not have it now. Dad's smoked turkey is now a tradition thing forever." I finished my bourbon as well and we called it a night.

Chapter 15

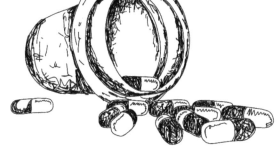

The smell of cinnamon, honey, and ham dominated the kitchen. The cat was sprawled out on her back sunbathing in the dining room where we had the curtains open. Liz was talking to Mom and managing the cooking in the kitchen. We had barbecued green beans, stuffing, mashed potatoes, potato salad, cream cheese bacon jalapenos, and three kinds of pie all being made in there. She was doing amazing work in there.

I continued walking through the kitchen and out back to the grill. The smell of smoky charcoal, turkey, and herbs hit me, "Oh my god, Dad... that smells amazing. Everything smells amazing right now. I can't wait to eat!"

"Dude, I tried to go get some bacon earlier and Liz swatted at me with the wooden spoon!" Donny threw a stick and his dog, Lula, took off after it like a rocket.

Joseph waggled a finger at Donny, "Don't fuck with Liz, man. She owns that kitchen right now."

Alex silently slunked his way over to me and set his head on my shoulder. "Hey, check this out." He rolled up his sleeve to reveal an intricate, gorgeous tattoo of a thorny vine with exotic flowers covering nearly the entire area of skin from his wrist up to his elbow. "I got it a while ago. I've been meaning to go get it colored in but haven't had the time."

I grabbed his wrist and gently pulled it closer, "Woah... dude, this is really good. Who did the art?"

One side of Alex's lips turned into a sly smile, and it formed a dimple in his cheek, "I did."

I was jealous of his drawing skill. "Dude, this is like, legit... really good..." I turned his arm, inspecting the design. "I kinda want a copy of the artwork." I wondered how he afforded such a large and beautiful tattoo. It wasn't done by an amateur tattoo artist either, so I know he paid some serious cash for it. I decided it was better to let that topic go on Thanksgiving.

"Okay boys," Dad opened the smoker, "I need someone to get me a big plate or a cookie sheet and some aluminum foil for this turkey. We're almost done!" He clapped his hands together.

"I got it!" Donny ran inside and Lula followed him.

There was so much more I wanted to talk about with Alex, but it was time to eat. I hoped that we'd get some more time before he left. Jack and Tiffany arrived, then we ate dinner. After dinner and dishes, we were all hanging out on the front patio and talking.

"Personally..." I started, "I think it would be so cool if we all pitched in and bought a bunch of land somewhere and built homes across the property. It'd be nice to have my own home, but still be close enough to everyone to get together for dinners or whatever as often as we wanted to." I let myself get pleasantly lost in that thought.

"I just want to own and run my own hydro shop." Donny added.

Joseph shrugged, "I'm okay with what I have right now. Things are pretty good." He smiled, reflecting. "I'm just happy I finally have my own place."

Dad looked between us, "I love you boys so much. I'm so proud of y'all."

I looked at the beer bottle in my hand and thought back to my teenage years.

"No! You think you're the God of my life or something." I protested loudly. "Like I should bow to all your wishes. It's my own life! Just because you're too dumb to understand what I wan-"

Dad shot up from his chair, using his massive size to intimidate

15-year-old me, "Boy!" He yelled in his deep drill instructor voice, "You live under -MY- roof! You will do what I say or you will find another place to live. Are we clear?" He was pointing a knife-hand in my face and holding his beer bottle in the other hand.

I scoffed, "So that's it then? Those are my two choices? Slavery or homelessness? Great ultimatum. Some Dad of the year you're going to be." I could appreciate now that I was kind of an ass about things back then, but so was he.

Dad's shoulders started heaving as he started breathing heavier and heavier, his eyes radiated with anger. "Boy, you have about 4 seconds to get to your room or I'm gonna beat your little ass so bad your own momma's not gonna recognize you." He hadn't stopped pointing the knife-hand at me.

I turned to walk off, "Fuck you, dick head." I said under my breath.

"WHAT, BOY?!" Dad nearly hit the ceiling.

I started forward and heard Dad take a couple quick steps after me. Oh fuck... I sprinted into the kitchen, and he chased me around the table. I was legitimately scared. Dad had already finished a few beers since he'd been home from work, and he was nearing the point of unreasonable anger. I had myself to thank for pushing him, but the situation was out of control now. I don't even remember the things we hollered at each other, but I remember running around and around the table until his beer bottle flew across the table, exploding against the wall in front of me.

I looked back at the beer bottle in my hand and around at my Dad and brothers. How did we get from there to here? I didn't know the answer to that question, but I could still appreciate the fact that things had certainly become better.

Dad had changed and become such an awesome person. It was for that reason that I now respected him most. It couldn't have been easy, but he never once complained about anything or put himself on display to receive praise. He simply did the hard work that was in front of him and became such an awesome person for it. That was an example worthy of following in my mind.

"I'm not feeling great, so I'm gonna go lay down now. Good cooking tonight everyone! Love you all!" Mom's voice was energetic and bubbly on the surface but had a layer of struggle beneath it. We could never tell when she was just trying to control our perception of her or when she really felt bad, so we just let her do whatever she wanted to do and didn't really have any expectations of her.

"All right, good night, Momma," Dad acknowledged her.

Jack looked at Dad, "So, what was the craziest thing you saw in your time in the Army?"

"Oh man…" Dad inhaled a puff of his cigarette, "I'd have to say the time I was transporting a nuclear warhead. There were 5 vehicles in my convoy. We got pulled over by a single cop. The cop ended up asking me to get out of the vehicle. He wanted to know what we were transporting in his county. I said, 'Officer, this is classified material, property of the US Military. You will not search these vehicles.' And you know, he was a young guy. Had a big ego. So he looked at me and said, 'You'll surrender to a search unless you want to be arrested for obstruction of justice.' And he just started walking over to the transport truck with the warhead.

So I put my hand on my sidearm, and my driver saw it and gets out. I shout at the officer, 'Sir, I highly suggest you take about 45 seconds and go call your superiors before you do something stupid." Dad stopped, taking another drag from his cigarette.

We all looked at Dad with anticipation, "What happened after that?" I asked for everyone.

"Well," Dad started, "When some of the other vehicles saw my driver get out, they got out too. I guess the cop looked around, saw my hand on my sidearm, saw my guys all there and he wisened up. He went back to his squad car, spent a few minutes on the comms, and came back apologizing and he let us go." Dad started laughing. "That guy almost fucked up big time."

Jack shook his head, "Jeez man… that's crazy. Don't you have to call those things in to the local police departments, so they know what's going on ahead of time?"

Dad nodded, "Yep. So, this guy either missed the meeting that morning or didn't pay attention, or something." Dad finished his beer, "And we were given explicit orders to shoot anyone who tried to tamper with it. It was a nuclear warhead, after all. I thought I was going to have to shoot a cop, man. That's not cool."

Jack winced, "Yeah man, that's a rough spot to be in. I don't envy that one bit."

"Well boys," Dad stood up, grabbing his two empty beer bottles, "It's time for this old man to go to sleep. I'm wiped."

"Yeah, I need to get the fam home. Thanks for the awesome food!" Jack stood up, too.

Everyone either left or went to bed for the night but Alex and me. I wondered if we were going to get an opportunity to talk. I wanted to know how he was doing because I never really had the opportunity to talk about anything that was actually going on in his heart and life. He loved to talk about aliens, or Alan Watt's theories, but never the cold hard reality of what was happening around us.

Alex's air mattress was set up back in my office, so we went back there and talked.

"Bud, how are you doing? You, on the inside, underneath the surface, and the small talk?" I sat down on the air mattress next to Alex and put my arm around him.

He shrugged, "I'm K. Life isn't happy, it's not sad. It just is."

I didn't really know how to process that, but I wondered if that was the methadone having an effect on him. "What about the girlfriend and the place you had with her? Weren't you at least a little bit happy during that?"

Alex shook his head, "No. That didn't make me happy. That made my life way more confusing." Alex laid down, "Come lay down next to me please?"

I laid down next to him, but the way he snuggled up to me made me feel incredibly uncomfortable. It made me feel just like I did when I was frozen as Samuel performed sexual acts on me. I tried to stay there in case it was just innocent, but I couldn't. It was keeping me in a bad head space, so I got up after a few moments and went to the bathroom.

When I walked back into the office, Alex had a big bottle of my allergy meds and he had dumped about 500 pills from it into a baggy. I caught him with the pill bottle in one hand and the open baggy in the other.

Startled, he spun around, "Oh hey." He tried to slyly slide the baggy under the air mattress.

I was already emotionally heightened from my own traumas, and I kind of snapped on him, "What the hell was that man? Are you stealing pills? What even are those?"

"Psh," He scoffed, "You're overreacting. Jeez. They're allergy pills, Lenny. I'm not gonna abuse allergy meds." He acted misunderstood and incensed.

"Man, give me those back. I don't know why you want a half-bottle of allergy pills, but you're not getting them from me." Now I was scared. One doesn't look for and steal a half bottle of allergy meds for no reason. I walked over and took them from him. To my surprise, he didn't resist at all.

Alex shook his head, "Why does everyone always overreact to everything? This is so stupid. I just wanted some allergy meds to take back up to Indiana with me."

"You could have asked, man. You didn't have to go behind my back and steal them from me." I realized I was feeling hurt that he would steal from me, so I tried to reason with him, hoping to connect with something. "Bud, what's going on?"

Alex shrugged, "What do you mean?"

I sighed. "Not these games again man... You know exactly what I mean."

Alex shrugged again, "I don't know what you're talking about."

"Ok, whatever." I put my hands up, "I'm going to bed. I can't stop you from stealing anything from me. Do whatever the hell you want." I was so frustrated. I was trying to honestly connect with him, and there he was stealing allergy meds from me. What the hell was going on? This felt weird. Of all the things he could steal, why allergy meds? And why in such a hurry?

I tried to enjoy the rest of the time that Mom, Dad, and Alex were there, but I suddenly didn't know where to place Alex in my life. I couldn't get that interaction out of my mind. I knew that he had stolen from Mom and Dad pretty often, but he had never stolen from me. A line had been crossed and trust had been breached. I'm pretty sure I was the only one who hadn't had their trust breached by him at this point, so I don't know why I was so surprised. I thought he loved me so much that he would never do something like that to me. It wasn't the allergy meds that mattered to me, it was the lying and the covering up of it afterwards that really got me.

Something was obviously wrong with Alex, but what? How could I help if he was keeping me at arms' length? I'd do anything for him, if I could just figure out what to do. Giving him money wasn't the answer because he'd just spend it all on Methadone or actual heroin. He didn't want to come stay with me and find a job and try to make something with himself. What more could I do? I felt stuck, with no clear solution in sight.

After they left for Indiana, I went back to my daily work routine. I couldn't really get that interaction with Alex out of my head though. I got home after the first day of work after Thanksgiving break and settled in, playing some video games to wind down before bed.

"Big incoming guys, big incoming!" I announced over Discord voice chat.

"I see 'em, get ults ready, let's head right into them!" Akinos gave the order.

My phone started ringing, "Ah, shit, I'm getting a phone call. Let me die, I need to AFK for a minute." I informed my friends in voice chat.

I saw it was Mom calling, so I stood up from my computer chair and answered it, "Hey Mom. What's up?" I started walking into the kitchen for a drink.

I couldn't hear anything, so I answered again, "Hello? Mom, you there?"

"Hey.. uh, hey, Sweetie." She sounded upset. "Are you sitting down?"

Uh oh, this doesn't sound good. Did their dog, Bandit die? Did Dad get fired? "No," I answered simply. "I'm getting some water. Why what's up? What's wrong?"

"Ummm, is Liz near you?" She asked.

"Oh my god, Mom, no, Liz's in our bedroom. What's up?" I couldn't stand the dramatic, ominous questions. "Just rip the Band-Aid off, whatever it is." I pleaded.

"No, honey, go get Liz and let me know when you guys are sitting down together." She definitely sounded like she'd been crying a good bit.

"Is Dad okay? Is everyone okay?" I was getting worried.

Dad's voice came through the phone, "I'm fine buddy, but go sit down with Liz." He sounded like he'd been crying, too.

Oh shit... what happened? I hurried into the bedroom with Liz, "Hey babe, Mom and Dad are on the phone. They asked me to come get you." I sat on the bed next to her and put the phone on speaker mode. "Okay, we're here, sitting on the bed. What's up?"

I heard Dad inhale and exhale several times, "Oh my god... this is so hard... Um..." Dad was trying to breathe and clear his throat. "Alex, uh..."

Oh no... oh no...

"Alex c-" Dad's voice started cracking, "About an hour ago. He-" Dad choked, "Alex committed s- suicide." He burst into tears.

"Oh no... no... no, no, no, no, no..." No other word came to mind. I started crying and panicking... looking around... for... what exactly? I slid off the bed and put my head in my hands, crumpling into the floor, "No, no, no, no..." This was the worst-case scenario. I thought I had time. "No, no, no, no..." My crying had quickly reached that point where you can't breathe and start choking on your own snot. I tried to open my eyes, but when I noticed almost no color, it made me sick to my stomach, so I just kept them closed. I coughed and cried, and coughed and cried some more. I had forgotten my entire vocabulary except the word "no".

Liz had gotten off the phone with Mom and Dad so they could call Donny and Joseph and give them the news. She sat with me on the floor for about 30 minutes before we called Mom and Dad back.

"Hey Buddy..." Dad answered his phone.

"Hey Dad," Liz greeted him for me. "We've cried a lot, but I think Len has some questions if you're okay with it?"

"I'll do my best." He sobbed.

"I love you, Dad." I started, then paused for thought.

"I love you too, buddy." Dad's voice was wobbly with emotion.

"How did he do it?" I asked as calmly as I could.

"He hung himself with..." Dad's voice trembled and cleared his throat, "with 550 paracord."

"Where?" I'd hoped I wasn't being rude to Dad, but I was desperately trying to piece Alex's last moments together.

"From his closet door." Dad started crying. I'd never heard that man cry before tonight, and now he couldn't stop.

I started to cry again, "How..." I swallowed the lump forming in my throat, "How'd you find him?"

"Your Mom just went in there to check on him. We hadn't heard anything from him in a couple of hours, and normally he's making food or going to the bathroom, or getting water, or something..." His voice trailed off in thought.

I had just managed to get my emotions somewhat under control when I started back into crying.

I got off the phone with Dad and spent the rest of the night trying to process things. I asked Liz to call Jack and see if he was able to come over, too. He came over, but I don't remember anything we talked about. I just remember the thoughts I was trapped in my skull with.

Gone... just... gone. No more hope that he could turn his life around and find happiness. No more getting excited when he spontaneously showed up for holidays. No more of his awesome artwork.

But also, he wouldn't be stealing jewelry from Mom and Dad anymore. He wouldn't be stuck in depression anymore. Dad would finally have a chance to pull ahead financially, because Alex wouldn't be taking every dime that wasn't promised to bills or food.

I thought about all the diapers I changed. I thought about baby Alex splatting me with spaghetti and giggling. I thought about all the hopes and dreams I had for my little brother.

It wasn't supposed to be like this... I was going to help Alex get his act together and he was going to be a success story. I guess I wasn't fast enough...

I wondered what he experienced in his last moments. Did he reach a point of regret and try to get down, but was stuck and couldn't call for help? My spine shivered. Was he even fully conscious for the process? Was he having a depressive episode and would have regretted it in a few days?

My thoughts turned inwards. How could I have been a better brother to make it worth it to him to stay here with us? Was the straw that broke the camel's back the way I snapped at him for stealing the allergy meds? Or did he have this planned and no amount of outside intervention could have prevented this?

Even after I had cried to exhaustion and Jack had left, I still couldn't sleep. Was there any kind of afterlife? Was there a way to see Alex again? I could acutely see now why religion was as powerful as it was.

I'd heard fringe theories of people proposing that human consciousness returns to Mother Earth after the body dies, or it goes to Heaven or Hell, or it gets reincarnated, or even that it crosses dimensions of time and space to find its next home. That all felt superficial and arrogant of me to assume, without any proof, that my consciousness lives on forever. I'd love to believe that my own consciousness is important to some esoteric function of the universe, but I simply couldn't find any evidence to support the idea.

I thought about the conversations I had with Alex when I'd visit him. Now, looking back, they were filled with talks of different afterlife theories. Was this the reason behind his fascination with the afterlife? How could I have missed it?

I remembered the abuse he suffered at the hands of the principal of the private Christian academy we went to. After I went off to college, Alex had been beaten badly by the principal of the Academy. Paddlings were a common occurrence, but Alex had gotten an attitude with the Principal. He paddled my little brother until he bled through the skin on his butt cheeks and lost control of his bowels. Alex was 9 years old then and I didn't find out until years later after I had gotten married and been living on my own. Did that trauma haunt him until he was driven to this? I wanted to go break that man's legs who did that.

My brain wouldn't stop with the questions. I almost had to talk myself into believing it was real. I had just seen him a day and a half ago...

Would I wake up from this nightmare soon?

Surreal...

Chapter 16

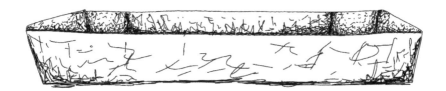

Two days later, I stared numbly into a cardboard box containing my little brother's body. A cardboard box? I'm not sure what else I expected, but it seemed so degrading. I guess that's life.

I pulled the collar of his jacket back and slipped a note into his jacket pocket, revealing the ligature marks around his neck. I never thought he'd ever do something like this. How could I not see this coming? If I were smarter or had paid more attention, maybe I could've prevented this...

I put my hand against his forehead. He was so cold. My eyes started tearing up and I choked on what I would have thought was charcoal if I weren't so familiar with swallowing my emotions. There used to be so much potential in this now lifeless body in front of me. It was both familiar and foreign at the same time. I stared at his closed eyes, getting lost at sea in my memories and emotions... my hand still feeling the cold forehead.

"Twins?!" I asked, making sure I heard Mom correctly. "I'm gonna be a big brother... like... twice?!" little 9-year-old me marveled excitedly.

Mom turned around in the front passenger's seat, "That's right! You're going to be a big brother... twice!" Mom put two fingers up and smiled at me with pure joy.

"OHHHH, this is so cool that this is happening to me! I'm gonna be the best big brother ever!" I bounced in my seat with excitement, triggering my seat belt lock. I stared out of the back seat window at the passing streetlights and let my imagination run wild with possibilities.

I wanted to show them how to ride bikes and rollerblade. I wanted to proudly introduce them to all my friends. I wanted to help them with their homework and beat up all their bullies with the karate I didn't know. Though I had no idea what I was doing, it gave me a sense of purpose and identity. It didn't matter that I had no clue, I'd learn whatever I needed to. I had to be there for them when they needed me.

I instantly understood back then that I could have a different relationship with them than Mom or Dad could, and I took that as a responsibility to give them the best version of that relationship I could. They were already the coolest little brothers ever, and I hadn't even met them yet. I had to live up to my end of that bargain and be the best big brother ever.

I blinked and wiped the tears away from my eyes and Alex's face came back into view. I was crying heavily by this point and trying to do it as quietly as possible. I didn't care if anyone saw me angry, but I couldn't let anyone see me cry in sadness. I didn't want someone to mistakenly think it was a public display for sympathy and come touch me. I looked back at the door to the viewing room and saw Mom sitting on the couch in the hallway relishing in the affection being poured onto her.

I closed my eyes and put my hand in my pocket. My hand found Liz's little ladybug and clenched it like a lifeboat in this emotional storm.

I toyed with Liz's ladybug in my hand. Joseph, Donny, and I stood in my Aunt's kitchen. We were surrounded by family I hadn't seen in at least 15 years.

"Len, what is going on with your Mom? She comes out here to Colorado last week, tells everyone how your Dad is abusing her back in Indiana, then goes into the emergency room. Can you give us any idea of

what's going on?" My Aunt Leigh asked.

"Wow..." I shook my head in disbelief "I don't know where that would come from. I know she wanted to move out to Colorado a couple months ago, but Dad told her they couldn't do it financially. I know she's been pretty mad about that, but he's the farthest thing from abusive to her. He takes care of her and she sleeps on the couch all day. She might get up and make a meal or vacuum if she feels like it, but 90% of her days are spent sleeping. Dad takes care of everything because she complains if she ever has to do something when she doesn't feel like it."

Aunt Jane raised her hand quizzically, "So, he's not abusing her in any way?"

Donny scoffed, "Hell no, but she'll spin a story up however she can to try to get people to pay her way out here through sympathy. Mom is addicted to her pain meds. You guys are dealing with an addict, so expect addict behavior. We've given up on trying to talk to her about doing anything differently because she just doesn't listen."

Aunt Leigh pointed at me, "Len, she cried for hours telling us how he was keeping her hostage and not letting her go do her doctor's appointments and forcing her to cook dinner after having a seizure. What the hell are we supposed to think?"

I pinched the bridge of my nose, "Oh my god... are you serious? We've been pissed at her for years because she's the one who constantly cancels her own doctor appointments. We've given up on it by now. And as for the hostage thing... we would all love it, Dad included, if she'd get off the couch and do something. It'd be even better if whatever she found to do got her out of the house for a change. She's the one keeping herself hostage, if anything. And come on, you guys all know who Mom is. Do you think anyone's going to force her to do anything she doesn't want to on a good day, let alone after a seizure?"

Aunt Jane's eyes softened, "You're not wrong about that."

I put my hands up defensively, "Now, full disclosure here, she has a bad UTI that she has let go for a long time and she's septic right now. That's why she's still in the hospital. So she could have been making shit up in a septic fever, too. But it is also one hundred percent in-character for *her to fabricate some emotional story to drum up some sympathy toward whatever goal she's working at. In this instance, it sounds like she's trying to get you guys to move her out here to Colorado because Dad told her no."*

I looked around before continuing, "You know, this isn't the first time she's done this either. When she moved to Indiana and took the boys with her, she came up on a vacation trip for some family reunion and put on the water works. The family up there bought into the sob stories she sold them and moved her and the boys up there from Memphis. They even gave her a place to stay, as long as Dad helped pay the rent up there. It took Dad two years to get the finances settled so he could rejoin his family. And he never complained once."

Aunt Leigh shook her head, "How did it get this bad with her?"

I dipped my head and shrugged.

I toyed Liz's ladybug in my hand again, watching Mom talk out in the hallway and Dad lightly rubbing her shoulder in comfort. I couldn't use my tears to garner sympathy and attention like she did, and I couldn't let anyone think that's what I was doing if I did end up crying. The only solution was to not be seen crying by anyone, ever. Then nobody would feel obliged to give me sympathy and I wouldn't feel weird about getting it. Sympathy was wasted on me anyway. What could anyone really do to make anything better? Alex was gone. No amount of kind words would fill the gaping void left in the fabric of my identity now.

"Goodbye, Alex." I leaned down and kissed his cold, pale forehead and left.

Alex was cremated later that afternoon and his remains were put in an urn for the memorial service. Four pounds of ash was all that remained of my little brother now. Life hit differently.

After Alex's memorial service, Joseph and Donny helped me clean up Alex's room. We probably should have called a hazmat team out to clean the room it was so bad, but we muscled our way through it.

I slid the glass sliding door open and the smell hit me like Mike Tyson. It smelled like hot funk. I took a careful step in, searching for a place to slide my foot between trash to reach the floor. The trash was almost up to my knee once

I stepped down fully into the room. There was no use. We were going to have to just start cleaning from the door.

It took us two full days to clean Alex's room. It was filthy. How had Alex lived like this? How could anyone live like this? Dad said that one of the main things they fought about was him cleaning up his room. And he always took hours to clean up when I was traveling on the road and would stop by. I guess it kinda made sense now.

Alex's bed was a fold-out couch bed. The arms and back of the couch were almost entirely covered with trash. The bed was entirely covered with trash. We found many empty water bottles filled with urine, thankfully with the caps tightened back on. Old fast food had been left in bags and squished under the weight of the rest of the trash above it. In one corner, he was planting a small tree and trying to bring it back to life. Dirt was all over in that corner.

And in the corner, next to the pile of dirt, was the closet. About 6 inches of 550 cord was still hanging from the clothes rod where the paramedics cut Alex down. This was right where Alex spent his last moments. If only I'd been right in this very spot 70 hours ago. I missed it by that much...

As we cleaned, I was still having a hard time coming to terms with things. Just a few days ago, he was safe right here... I reminded myself he was gone and I'd never see him again. I weathered a wave of disbelief and nausea before my brain was back in line with reality.

After 3 days off work and a weekend up there, we had to get back home and back to the grind. I was kind of shell-shocked driving home. So that was it then? This whole thing was over now and life would just continue like normal?

I couldn't remember much of anything that anyone said to me during that trip. I was trapped in my own skull with my own thoughts again. No amount of telling myself not to think about things too much was proving helpful. I simply didn't have that level of strength over myself now. I knew something happened to me inside, but I didn't know what. I had to figure it out again...

I decided to use my time during the trip to think about my life real hard. I thought about my life back home. About all the things I wanted to be different. I spent so much time working and not enough time with the people I loved. I had myself to blame for that. The worst part of it, I blew a lot of the money I was making. Once I paid off my debts and got to a good place financially, I just spent more money. I didn't save anything. I had nothing to show for that time except some paid off debt and a sports car that cost me way too much money. None of that did Alex any good. I had failed Alex as a big brother in a way that I didn't fully understand.

Suddenly all those flashy things that I thought were important to me seemed completely irrelevant. I'd take the debt back and trade the sports car for Alex, but unfortunately reality doesn't work that way. I seemed to be butting heads with reality more and more.

Alex was gone, but Donny and Joseph were still here. It may have been too late to do anything about Alex, but what could I learn from this and apply to Donny and Joseph to minimize any future regrets with them? My previous resolve regarding not thinking too much about life was also crumbling. Did I really believe it was best to nonchalantly disregard the things that bothered me? Weren't those supposed to be some indicator of where I can improve my life?

Once I got back to work, life wasn't the same. I felt both exposed and invisible in the worst ways. I loved teaching my team before, but now I just viewed my team under me as energy vampires. I wasn't getting the satisfaction that I used to out of teaching others, and it was just an energy sink. It was something that now took an insurmountable amount of energy to maintain, and I felt like nobody could see that to appreciate how much energy this took now. I had my legs swept out from under me and everyone around me just expected me to be the same as I'd always been to them. But I knew I wasn't the same. The depression was back in full force, and I felt like it was on display for the whole office to see and silently judge. I hated being in the office.

I had been slowly worked into more and more responsibilities and consistently lied to about plans to be fairly compensated. I had been led on for years this way. Why was I holding onto hope that anything would ever change with that situation? It wouldn't ever change because that model was working for everyone above me, they just had to put up with some complaining from me every few months.

I was not feeling very patient toward work anymore. I found the whole situation to be tragically typical. I approached Francis one day looking for a solution.

"Francis, you got a minute?" I said knocking on his open door.

He looked up from his laptop, "Of course, come on in."

I shut the door behind me, "Hey man, I need some help. I know you've been working on getting me put into a role with the right pay, but honestly, I don't want that anymore. I want to come in, put in my 8 hours a day and go home like a normal job. I need to achieve some kind of balance in my life right now man." I pleaded.

He shook his head, "That's not how this industry works, Len. I don't have the luxury of choosing our hours. We have to keep up with the workload or the work goes to someone else, and then we have no business at all."

"I understand," I put my hand up in acquiescence, "But I don't want the lifestyle that you expect from your leadership. You expect the leadership to be sold out for the business, and that's not unreasonable, but that's also not where I'm at right now. I need something a lot less stressful. I want to go back to just doing the responsibilities of my actual title I was hired in as and still have. I just want to be an engineering assistant. I'm still not even at the cap for that pay bracket, so I wouldn't go down in pay at all." I hoped it was clear that I had put some thought into this and I was serious about it.

Francis's face contorted with frustration and his skin flushed red, "Damnit Len, I've been working on getting you into this position because you've been on my ass for a very long time about it. Don't waste my fucking time!" He was yelling by the end of that.

I felt the tingle of anger instantly start moving up the back of my neck. I wanted to ask him why his time was the only time that he cared about wasting. I wanted to ask him why he never took me seriously. I wanted to remind him that I can only put up with being lied to for so long before I give up hope.

I refrained from saying anything in response ultimately because I knew there was a high likelihood of some kind of emotional reaction if I started down that road. I didn't want to start crying and lose my shit in the office. I simply left Francis's office with a firm understanding that I could not look to him as a friend who would help me find a solution. He was a boss trying to keep the money flowing in and that was it.

I kept my headphones in as long as I could, hoping the folks under me would just figure things out without me. It was hard to think. I'd stare at a set of work prints and it meant nothing to me. The only thing that mattered was this cloud of sadness I was stuck in that didn't seem to matter to anyone but me.

But I also found out that Francis took a donation from the office to help pay for Alex's memorial service costs, and I'm pretty sure he put the majority of funds into that. Joseph and Francis had developed a good friendship, so I figured he did that for Joseph, not so much for me. Francis acted like my friend in a lot of ways except where it impacted my life the most. It was confusing and made me feel manipulated.

My mind was made up though. I didn't want a leadership position anymore. I knew I would just continue to be abused. I just didn't have the energy for all that anymore. I just wanted to work my 8 hours and focus on writing. I wanted to publish a book during my off time and work toward independence so I could quit this job eventually.

But I couldn't get enough time away from work to do anything. I was still being subtly forced into working a ton of extra time because I knew I'd get in trouble if I left before all the work was finished. This is when suicidal thoughts entered the picture.

I drove into work one morning. Joseph had let me borrow his truck while he was out of town, so thankfully I didn't have to use the motorcycle today since it was raining. About 2 minutes from pulling into the parking lot, I got overwhelmed with emotions and started crying. I made it to the parking lot out front of work, but I couldn't stop crying. And it was escalating. I felt like I was going to die. My heart was racing. I had to get in to work, but I couldn't force myself to stop crying and get out of the truck. I was a mess.

But what the hell was I going to do now? Tell Francis I couldn't work today because I was upset? I wanted to implode out of existence.

I texted Jerry, who was now my immediate manager. "I can't come into the office man." I sent him the text. I was crying and heaving. He came outside, drove me around the block a couple times, and he talked me down. I eventually calmed down and went in to work, but I was not very productive at all. I was tired all day and just didn't want anyone to talk to me.

A few weeks later, during the coldest part of January, I was driving home on my motorcycle after another long day of work. It was dark and I had started crying about half-way home. This was not good because my tears and snot were freezing inside my helmet as I was driving. My visor was also fogging up pretty bad because my breathing was heavy. I just had to make it home...

By the time I made it home, I was so worked up with fear, sadness, frustration, and suicidal thoughts that I was shaking. I rolled up my driveway. I could see the parking spot for my bike at the end of the driveway and tried to focus on that. I barely got my kickstand down in time and turned to rush inside the house. I was breathing like I'd just run a marathon and felt a little lightheaded on top of all the emotions. I felt hot and couldn't breathe. But I was bundled up and strapped for safety. There was a long process to putting on and removing my winter riding gear. I tried dumbly removing my helmet, but my brain wasn't functioning correctly in that moment. It was a whole-head helmet and the chin strap was tightly secured, so I was just ultimately tugging on my lower jaw. The shakes grew even worse and I let out a pathetically weak, primal, growlish-moan as my knees wobbled.

My headphones underneath my helmet blasted Slipknot at the loudest volume, "I'm gonna suffer for the rest of my life, but I will always find a way to survive. I'm not a failure but I know what it's like. I can take it or leave it or die." I'd heard those lyrics a thousand times before, but they hit differently in this moment, stumbling toward my house.

I couldn't get my helmet off, so I tried to get my backpack off. With my 2 layers of riding gloves still on, I didn't have the dexterity to unbuckle the plastic clasp across my chest that held my backpack securely in place. I pulled my arms up and inward, grabbing the straps at my chest. I gave the hardest heave I could force to break the plastic clip and I felt it give. I stumbled, but worked the backpack off one shoulder. As I fell to my back, I got the other shoulder free of the backpack straps and flung it as far as I could in whatever direction was away from me. I slammed into the ground, my backpack flying the other direction.

I laid there, breathing heavily, and crying. Why was my life instantly turning into such a tragic shit show? I hated everything about this. After a few minutes of lying there, crying and breathing, I came to my senses enough to take my gloves off and start unbuckling and unclasping things, but I was still manic.

I opened my visor and removed my glasses first, then my helmet. Each piece got flung out into the yard as it was removed. And with each piece of gear

I removed, I could breathe a little easier. I stripped down to my single layer of jeans and a t-shirt and laid in the pile of protective gear.

I noticed Liz standing there. How long had she been standing there? I looked at her with some frozen tears in my eyes and some frozen snot covering my beard in a cone that widened from my nose down to my chin, covering my beard and mustache. I started crying again once I noticed her, but now I was crying in defeat instead of frustration. I was the definition of a mess.

Chapter 17

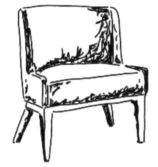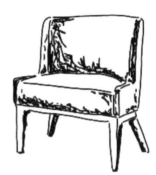

"I was up above it!" Trent Reznor's familiar voice blasted across my headphones, "Now I'm down in it!"

I'll never get to talk to Alex again... Fuck, I'd give anything to have him back. I just miss him so much... Why can't I function? Life sucks, and I kind of wish I believed in a supreme being so I could be mad at someone who was responsible for all this.

My heart was racing, I was holding my head in my hand at my desk, and bouncing my leg up and down rapidly. I was always right on the edge of tears, though I hoped no one could see that. I was hyper fixated on making sure I didn't let myself cross that line and cry in the office, though everything inside seemed to be pushing toward it.

"Hey Len... You okay?" I barely heard my name over my headphones.

I removed a headphone and looked up. "Hm? Yeah, I'm fine. What've you got?" I tried my best to be present and sincere, but I just wasn't. I hated the attention. I just wanted them to give me the problem so I could give them a solution and we could get the transaction over with. Why weren't they able to find their own solutions? I was so tired and sad. So sad and tired of it.

Luc looked at me with concern, but continued, "Okay, well... this project you assigned me to this morning... I just got the prints from Offshore, and they're all wrong."

I pushed my glasses up and pinched my nose, "The prints that are due to the customer today?"

He hesitated, "... yeah, those ones. But, there's more."

I turned my head and looked at him, pleading for mercy.

"Offshore did all the cable counts and distributions per the customer's old standard." He stated simply.

"Old standard?" I questioned. "There's a new one?"

Luc nodded, pleased with himself, "It came in just a few hours ago."

My eye twitched. "How do they expect us to keep up with their due dates if they keep changing the rules on us at the last minute?" I plopped my forehead onto my desk and wanted to blink out of existence.

I don't know how I missed that update though; it was my job to stay on top of those things... Usually, I did a good job, but it was getting harder and harder to focus. Seemingly small slippages like this added momentum to the depression and anxiety.

Luc was still standing there, waiting patiently for some marching orders.

I lifted my head, "Ok, uh... Hell I dunno, customer is either going to get it on-time and wrong, or late and correct. Screwed either way. I'll handle the email to the customer about this, but go ahead and mark it up with the corrections needed. Send it to Offshore by the end of your day today and tell them to have it back to us no later than noon tomorrow. Make sure you CC all the managers, too. We can't deliver it incorrect."

This job had so many moving parts. It was hard to keep up with it on an average good day, let alone with all this emotional crap piled on top.

I was painfully aware that I was in an unsustainable situation, but what was I supposed to do? Things just worked a certain way before and suddenly they didn't work that way anymore. Like if someone swapped our laws of physics out for completely new and even weirder ones.

The little things that brought me motivation just didn't anymore. I used to love teaching people. I found it incredibly satisfying. But now, I didn't want people to even look at me. In the past, I took it as a personal challenge to conduct myself like a good leader, but suddenly I felt that everyone should leave me alone and find their own way. I knew I had changed, but didn't know to what extent.

It wasn't just my work life where I saw the changes, though.

Jack came over and hung out with me at my place that night.

"Dude!" Jack was excited, "I can't wait for this weekend. It's gonna be great. All these people are gonna be there at my place."

I lit a joint, "Man, I gotta be honest. I'm not really feeling the big drinking parties anymore. I still want to hang out with you and Tiffany, but I just don't have the capacity for all the extra right now."

"Aw, don't worry about it. You're fine. It'll be good. You'll have fun." He jovially pressed.

I didn't want to argue. It was apparent that he wasn't listening. He thought he knew what was best for me, and I really felt like it was an honest mistake. He cared for me, but I did wish he'd listen. I wondered if I could approach it from a different angle. "Oh dude, what about some Elder Scrolls Online? You've been an Elder Scrolls fan forever, and it's a ton of fun. Liz, Tiffany, you, and me could do veteran dungeons together and do like a regular gaming thing!" I had just thought of the idea and was legitimately excited by it.

Jack soured a little, "Ehhhh, I just don't think I can get into video games man. I'm too busy. I've got too much going on."

I frowned. Too busy for video games, but not too busy for hours-long parties on the weekend? That sounded like an excuse to me. "Dude, what? Not into video games? Do you realize how little sense that makes to me right now?" Jack and I talked about video games all the time.

Jack bobbed his head back and forth, "No like, I mean..." He paused, collecting his thoughts, "I dunno, I like single player games man. I don't really like multiplayer games."

I shrugged, "Ok, I guess that makes a certain amount of sense." I gave up. It did make a little bit of sense, but not completely. It didn't matter though, it was apparent he didn't want to play video games for whatever reason.

We hung out some more that night and talked, but not about anything in particular. Aliens, politics, nuclear energy, the usual suspects. But I was changing and I had no idea how to get that across to Jack. I know he just wanted things to be like they used to be, but I didn't want those things anymore. I still wanted his friendship, but I wanted a change of lifestyle that he didn't want.

After Jack left, I tried to get to sleep but couldn't. After a couple hours of tossing and turning in bed and being frustrated, I got back up and went back to the office. Was I somehow wrong or bad for changing? Was this what losing one's mind looks like from the inside? I was tired of the college party atmosphere that Jack and I had been living in the last few years. It seemed so superficial now that Alex was gone. How could Jack not see that? Why did that make me feel so invisible?

Lost in my thoughts, I wandered into the kitchen. It was still a wreck from last weekend's party. I surveyed the damage. Dried whiskey and barbecue sauce splotched the island counter randomly. A sinkful of dishes marinaded in cold, soapy water. Everyone went home and this was my payment for hosting a good time? I'd let it sit for 4 days because I was too busy trying to lick my emotional wounds while I was at home. The dirty house didn't help with the depression though, and I knew it. I wasn't OCD by any means, but I knew that I'd always felt better in a cleaner environment. The warzone that I called a kitchen was a problem though.

I couldn't find the motivation to clean it last weekend, and I knew I'd probably push off cleaning until a few hours before the next party, just like I had done the time before that and before that. But there wouldn't be a next party for me. The thought of cleaning my house and it staying clean was legitimately exciting, and since very little excitement pierced the shroud around me, I pursued it in the moment and cleaned the kitchen at 2 AM. I had work the next day, but I couldn't sleep anyway, so screw it.

While I did the dishes, I started re-evaluating all of my relationships to determine if I wanted to continue to put effort into them. I wished I could have taken all that time and effort I put into all those surface level relationships and instead found some way to funnel that energy toward Alex. Maybe he would still be here...

I was brought up to treat others as you would like to be treated. So I would treat everyone with the level of care and sincerity I would like to be treated with. My mistake was in also assuming that others would understand this behavior and reciprocate it. I remembered all the times I would spend $120 on food for one evening for 12 people, the same amount in alcohol, hours preparing and cleaning, and it just made me feel used. Nobody ever stayed to help clean or offered to help pay for food. Sometimes, people would bring their preferred bottle of liquor with them, but it wasn't all the time.

I finished cleaning the kitchen around 4:30 AM and made some coffee. I was still emotionally wired and not even remotely sleepy though, which I thought was good because if I fell asleep now, there's no way I'd wake up in an hour and a half for work. Francis wouldn't want to hear any of this nonsense about being kinda sad or tired, he just wants me to show up and suffer through it so we can keep the dollars flowing. I encouraged myself in the words of my favorite superhero, "Maximum effort, Len."

The energy and willpower it took to go to work each day was growing greater and greater. I felt so vulnerable in that huge single room with 40 other people in it. I wanted to not be seen, and I was forced to stay in an environment that was exactly the opposite. I literally didn't make eye contact with people anymore because I didn't want people to look at me for fear they might see the rot inside.

Francis wasn't letting me away from any of the extra responsibilities that had been packed on though, especially my leadership duties. So I approached him thinking I could have a conversation with him about the problem and find a possible solution.

"No." Francis said, shaking his head from side to side dramatically, "Absolutely not. Never. That will never happen as long as I am in charge." He sounded vehemently against the idea.

I sighed, "But dude... this doesn't make any sense to me. I can do my job just as effectively from home." I pleaded. How would I explain to him what was happening when I didn't even understand it? I couldn't.

But he was vehemently against it. I had my theories as to why, but they were just theories. I ultimately had no clue. I left his office and went back to my desk, put my headphones in, and continued to suffer through my workday.

A few days later, I snapped on him. I had just finished reading an email about a new sector of business that Francis wanted me to oversee. There was no way in hell I was letting him push me into more responsibilities. I didn't even care about the money anymore.

I sent him a pretty heated email and left one of my subordinates on the email chain. Francis came unglued that I would say what I said to him with a subordinate seeing the same thing.

"What the fuck is wrong with you, Len?" Francis shouted at me in his office.

"Maybe years of dealing with your bullshit is one of the things wrong with me. Did you consider that?" I snapped back. It was unusual for me to snap like this, and I recognized it.

Francis shook his head, "Len, get help. Have you looked into taking a leave of absence and seeing a therapist?"

I hadn't, but my ego was still too inflamed to be reasonable, "Have -YOU- considered seeing a therapist?" I retorted like a junior-high schooler. We were both being an ass, but he did have a point.

"You know, Len, nobody cares if you're right if you're an ass about it." He said condescendingly.

"If that's really true, then why does Jordan still work here? He's an even bigger ass than Chris is." I shot back.

Francis squinted in disbelief, "Oh whatever. Jordan's not an ass."

I nodded my head upward sarcastically, "Mmmm, ok. If you say so."

Francis shook his head, "Len go back to work."

The irony of two people, acting like asses to each other, also telling each other that nobody listens to assholes, was not lost on me. Interactions between Francis and I had been getting worse and worse.

He was right about one thing though; I really should go see a therapist. Especially after that weird incident on the motorcycle... That was definitely not normal.

I talked it over with Liz and she agreed it could be a good thing. So the next day, I applied for a leave of absence and set up my first therapist appointment. My leave of absence was approved by corporate almost immediately that same day. They weren't going to pay me for the duration, but I had been told that our insurance does provide options for paying me while I'm on LOA. I submitted all the paperwork for that to the insurance that day too.

It was almost surreal that I wouldn't have to come to work tomorrow. That happened so fast it was almost hard to believe. All the problems I had with work, suddenly gone. I could breathe. Things were looking up for a change. I slept for 12 hours straight that night.

I had gotten lucky with my therapist, because the first one I found was a hit, and I knew it from the first meeting I had with him later that week. I thought I was going to have to rifle through lots of therapists before I found one I resonated with.

"Hey! I'm Dr. Fulwiler." The man in front of me smiled pleasantly. He was only maybe an inch or two shorter than me, he had long hair that he wore in a ponytail, and glasses.

"Hey Dr. Fulwiler, I'm Len." I returned the formalities and we shook hands.

He waved me on, "Come on back to my office. Let's get to know each other a little bit."

We walked back to his office and he motioned toward a comfy looking chair, "Have a seat. I'll just start off by grabbing some basic info."

He took all my general information and recorded it in a document on his computer. After some brief surface level introductions, he spun his chair around and rolled it a few feet away from his desk. "So what brings you to see me today?"

I didn't know where to start. "I guess, uh... the shortest answer to that is depression and anxiety. But I don't want any prescriptions." I waved my arms in front of me, "Like, none at all. I need to be able to solve this through choice somehow."

Dr. Fulwiler smiled, "I think you've come to the right place. While I can prescribe medications if I have to, I don't like doing it unless there's no other option. I specialize in cognitive behavioral therapy. Basically, what that means is that we examine situations to find better ways to respond to emotions."

"Ok," I nodded excitedly, "That sounds exactly like what I'm looking for."

I told him about Alex and my problems at work. I told him about everything going on in my life and my previous struggles with depression. He helped me identify that the motorcycle incident and the time I cried in the parking lot at work were panic attacks. I honestly had no clue that's what a panic attack was. I just thought I was being an emotional nutcase and had to kick myself in the ass until I got over it.

In truth, I had no idea how to think about my emotions. As a male, I always felt the expectation to never let my emotions show. Other males historically ended up looking at me like something was wrong with me when I did - like I was giving the rest of the male population a bad name or something by being so shamefully human.

Dad and I didn't talk about emotional things. We talked about grilling techniques, our favorite brand of cigar or liquor, or old military experiences, but never emotions. As far as I could tell, there was some unspoken rule of manhood which stated you don't talk about your feelings. Dad told us he loved us and gave us hugs, and I'm thankful for that, but we never really talked about anything.

I ended up settling into one hour of therapy per week with Dr. Fulwiler. I'd keep notes of my experiences throughout the week and bring up anything I wanted to in the next session. I began noticing benefits from this immediately. This is exactly what I had been searching in the dark for all this time while telling myself I had to "figure it out". But what Dr. Fulwiler showed me was not what I thought I would find.

It was a process that took a long time, but he taught me how to identify my emotions when they would surface. He taught me that while I cannot necessarily control the emotions themselves, I can control my response to them. Identifying when a given emotion was present took a long time for me because it was an exercise in sitting through an emotional episode as an observer and not reacting at all to it. That's not something that came naturally to me.

He taught me to breathe my way through anxiety episodes as a way to control my heartrate. He taught me that I have many more options than I usually believe I do in an emotional moment.

Chapter 18

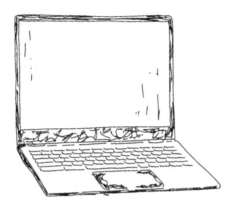

The same day I had that first meeting with my therapist, I reconnected with JP and Ingram through Discord. I had deactivated my Facebook account nearly 8 years ago, so Discord was my only social media account. I loved it that way. I could stay in contact with the people I wanted to and avoid all the crazy shenanigans on Facebook.

I told JP and Ingram all about Alex and how I was going to therapy now. They invited me to join them for their Friday night game nights as a way to escape and hang out.

This was just what I had been trying to get Jack and my brothers to do with me. It made me sad, but I knew if they wanted to come play video games with me, they would. I needed to manage my expectations better.

I joined JP and Ingram the following weekend, and it was so much fun. At the time, they were playing Overwatch. I wasn't ever interested in the game, but the game itself didn't matter so much as did the idea of a weekly game night. JP gifted the game to me so I could play with them.

"Awwww man... thank you dude, you didn't need to do that..." I said through Discord voice chat. I just noticed the pop up that I received a gifted copy of Overwatch from JP on Battle.net.

JP cackled victoriously, "No man, it's okay. I really want you to come play with us and not have to wait another two weeks to get paid. I'd do it again in a heartbeat. Anyway, Len, meet Luci and Thomas. I met Luci at work and we started doing game nights on Friday nights... what, maybe a year or so ago, right Luci?"

A female's voice chimed through Discord, "Damn skippy! It's been a hoot ever since." I could hear a bit of sarcastic humor in her tone and felt like I fit right in. "But yeah! So I'm Luci and this is my husband Thomathy."

"WHAT?! WHERE?!" Thomas shouted, "THAT MOTHER FUCKER OWES ME MONEY!"

Discord erupted in laughter.

Overwatch had finished downloading, so I launched it. "Alright, I'm in. What do I do? How dis game work?" I said in a silly tone. I was surprised that I felt good enough to be silly. I wanted to lean into that feeling.

"Oh! I see ya. Here, take this party invite..." JP said.

"Ok," I clicked to accept the invite and joined the party.

"Now I'll do this... and this..." I saw nothing happening on my screen, "... and we're off! Pick a hero!" The screen changed as JP spoke.

I was looking at a screen full of heroes, "Ok, who does what?"

They explained all the heroes to me, I made my choice, and we were off into our first match.

"Oh my god! What do I do? Ahhh!" I died.

"NOT MY ASSHOLE, NOOOO!" Thomas died too.

Discord erupted in laughter again.

"It's fine, we're fine. Ingram and Luci did some amazing healing and we saved the point, but hurry back!" JP was sort of our team leader. He played Overwatch semi-professionally for about a year, so I trusted him to lead us to victory.

"On my way back!" My role was to help protect the group from enemy damage by using my shield, but I had to be there to do my job.

"ONI-CHAAAAAAAN," Thomas was right behind me.

More unanimous laughter filled my headphones.

"Incoming!" Ingram said as we arrived.

I rounded the corner just as the enemy did. I used my ultimate ability out of reflex and stunned 4 out of 5 of their team members in one hit. JP followed up with his ultimate and we finished 4/5 of their team off. Thomas chased down the last one, hooked him back, and murdered him.

"Damn, Len and JP, save some ass for the rest of us!" Luci complimented us. We drank and gamed for hours that night. It was so much fun. It was downright therapeutic for me. Not the drinking part, but the gaming and hanging out part.

I was addicted to it. It became something I could be excited about all week. It had depth that weekend drinking escapades didn't in that I could plot and plan for what we would do for our Friday game nights. We played Overwatch, we played Dungeons and Dragons through Tabletop Simulator, we tried new games, and sometimes we just hung out and each played individual games.

Those three months that I was on my leave of absence went by so fast. I learned something during that time though. If I quit smoking weed and tightened my budget, which I had to do, Liz and I could make ends meet on her income alone. Ashamed because that meant that I had basically been pissing away my whole paycheck for years, I also felt empowered to realize that I could use my job purely to save money.

So when I got back to work, that's what I did. I had a new plan. I was going to save every dollar I made from work from now on and when I had enough to quit and do something different, I would do just that. That felt good.

When I got back to work, Francis had changed things up a bit...

Francis smiled pleasantly, "Hey! There he is!" He greeted me excitedly with a handshake and a pat on the back.

I smiled awkwardly, "Hey. How's things?" I asked, trying to be natural. I felt weird being back in the office though. I had identified that I had social anxiety in therapy. That vanished overnight as soon as I was able to be at home all the time, but it was rearing its head again now and I had nearly forgotten about it.

"So, Frontier is pretty slow right now and I've got it handled. I'm going to put you on Chris's team..."

I shot Francis a worried glance.

"... just for a little bit! I just need you there until Frontier picks up again." He assured me.

On the one hand, I was extremely thankful he wasn't putting me back into a position of leadership. On the other hand, he was putting me under Chris. That's what they did to Jack when they wanted him gone, too. There were 3 other managers that could have benefitted from me just as much as Chris. "Ok. That's no problem." I responded calmly. "I did want to be sure to talk to you about something specific though. My therapist and I both agree that I need to achieve some balance in my life. I can't work a bunch of overtime anymore. I simply can't. I will give it hell for the 8 hours a day that I can afford to give to Cyient, but I can't give anything beyond that."

"Oh yeah, sure, sure. Of course." I got the feeling Francis didn't hear a word I said.

I reported to Chris's office. "Hey Chris," I knocked on his open door.

"Hey Len," He said jovially in his thick southern accent, "Come on in."

I inhaled for patience and stepped in, "Francis just told me I'm under you for a bit. Whatcha need me doing?" I wanted to get right to business to minimize the opportunity we had to have a poor interaction. I'd seen enough of Chris's behavior that I did not respect him at all. I didn't respect him as a leader, and I didn't respect him as a person. This was something that took an enormous amount of self-control for me to keep my mouth shut around him and just be amicable.

"Aw," He waved his hand dismissively, "It's not much at all. It's nice and chill. I know you like chill." Was he trying to connect with me? "I've just got some AT&T service order work. Service order comes in, we design a path to the address they give us from the nearest splice point. Easy-peasy. Go see Devin, he'll get you set up."

Phew... that was fast and easy. "Sounds good, thanks man." I left his office and pursued my new role.

A few weeks in, we had an influx of service orders. I stayed 30 minutes late, breaking my commitment to myself, but ultimately realizing it wasn't a big deal. This was still way less than I'd worked in the past. After finishing up, I saw we had another service order come in. The two other folks who worked with me were gone already, but I had already stayed 30 minutes past my limit and went home.

I ran outside, got in Liz's Juke, and went to pick her up from work. She had been waiting on me to get off for about 30 minutes herself. We planned around our schedules to make sure we got off at the same time so we could share the Juke. I didn't want to ride the motorcycle after that panic attack, so we dealt with the logistics of sharing a car again.

I picked Liz up and we got some Little Caesar's on the way home and were eating the breadsticks in the car like the heathens we are. My phone started ringing.

"Hello?" I answered it.

"You left?" Chris asked.

"Yeah. I had stayed 30 minutes over already to finish one job. I'll get on that job that just came in first thing in the morning man." I answered him as matter-of-factly as I could.

"Nope. It doesn't work like that, Len. You don't leave if there's work still in the hopper." He sounded slightly irritated.

I inhaled for patience, "Chris, I told Francis when I started back working again that I was sticking to a 40-hour work week, at the suggestion of my therapist. This is something I'm doing for my own health. I will bust my ass for the time I am there, and I'll even stay 30 minutes late every now and then to finish up something I'm working on, but the days of me staying all night at work until I can't keep my eyes open, those days are done." I understood that he would probably feel like I was speaking out of turn, but I wasn't going to let myself get pushed back into the overworked craziness. I also expected there'd be some drama around it at first, until Francis and Chris got used to it.

"Wrong again, Len. I'm writing you up." He said with forced authority.

"Do what you gotta do man. Have a great night." I said sarcastically.

"Yep, see you in the morning." He said and hung up.

I relayed the conversation to Liz, but I only had to piece a few things together for her. She could hear most of it.

Liz squinted, "So, the job came in at 4 PM, and you have 24 hours to get it to the 1st step?" She was making sure she understood the process and handed me a piece of crazy bread.

"Yep." I took the breadstick.

"Why does he want you to do it tonight?"

I stuck the piece of crazy bread in my mouth and shrugged.

"If you send it in the morning, nothing is impacted right?" She started chewing on her breadstick too.

I swallowed, "Correct. Not a damn thing. What about the ones that come in at 6:30PM or 8 PM? They have to wait and nobody cares. The orders don't stop getting generated. Sometimes we come in to 2 or 3 orders in the morning, sometimes we come in to 10." I took another bite.

Liz shook her head, "I'm sorry you have to put up with these clowns."

I shrugged and swallowed after a moment, "It's fine. It's probably some testosterone-fueled power play." I attempted my best impression of a neanderthal, "ME SHOW HIM WHO BOSS. YOU NO TELL WHEN WORK. ME TELL WHEN DO STUFF." I beat my chest, "He's a jerk to people, and now I'm inside his insecure bubble of petty dominations." I realized I was being pretty judgy about Chris, but he'd earned it honestly.

The next day at work did, in fact, suck. I had never been written up at this job. Not once. Until today. And it was silly. Chris classified it as job abandonment. I wanted to break his legs again.

Why the hell was I working for this place? I ran a whole section of our business for 4 years, and Chris wants to get stupid and petty with my permanent work record? Oh right, I was working for this place because I really didn't have much other choice. Any other given business was highly likely to have unqualified dickheads for leaders too. At least I knew who the resident dickhead was here. I just had to get out from under him.

I had forgotten to breathe during the tense interaction where I had to sign that silly document, so by the time I left his office I ran straight out to the car. I could feel a panic attack coming on and I had to get alone. I felt hot and nauseous. I felt trapped in this job and in life and I wanted to die. Suicidal thoughts had me at their mercy. I was in tears for the better part of 20 minutes out there in my car. It made me feel like I had been specifically placed in a position to fail. I'd seen how they treated Jack when they wanted him gone. This was that same behavior. I chain smoked a few cigarettes, calmed down, and finished my day.

The very next day, Francis had to announce that we were closing the office for a couple weeks for this COVID thing that had just started popping up. That means everyone in the office had to transition to working from home. I found that to be cosmically hilarious. As we all know, the COVID-19 pandemic ended up lasting much longer than just a couple weeks.

Working from home was perfect for me. Francis moved me out from under Chris and gave me my own team again. I was thankful to be out from under Chris, but not so thankful to have the old leadership ropes back. But I could run it differently this time, and I would. I could still view my employee's screens and answer questions through remote software just as easily as if I were standing at their desk. I much preferred this new digital way of doing it. It made perfect sense to me for our industry.

And it worked well. It took a couple weeks for everyone to get situated, but I did a morning call with my team every morning at 8AM. I wanted to see coffee in their hands, I wanted to see their hair combed, and I wanted to see them ready for work. And they didn't disappoint.

My team worked 8 hours a day and went home. I'd managed to make it work not just for me, but for everyone on my team. Once we'd proved what we could do, I relaxed and didn't require the morning meetings or for them to be dressed as though we were working in the office still. If someone didn't come online by 9, I would text them and just make sure they were fine. They could make up any missed time from being late by working a little over. Things functioned well.

My therapist started doing remote sessions too, so even that was easier now. I was so happy I didn't purchase a car and instead shared the Juke with Liz for that little bit before the pandemic hit. I didn't need a car at all now and I was able to save so much more money because of it.

My weekly Friday game nights were still going strong, too. And that, in its own way, was a form of therapy too. I just enjoyed it so much.

A year and a half went by like this. I know the pandemic wasn't a good time for a lot of people, but for me, in my specific circumstance, I thrived in this new environment. I kept saving up money, working, doing therapy, playing games with my friends, and staying the hell away from people. Life finally felt sustainable. I was slowly but surely climbing out of the emotional pit I had fallen into.

I knew better how I had to deal with my own emotions now, so I was growing less and less patient for drama. Working from home, I had been blissfully unaware of the usual drama from work. It just vanished overnight when we all started working from home. In the complete absence of work drama, I'd lost any kind of tolerance to it. But something serious had been brewing while I worked from home.

Francis called everyone into the office for a meeting one day. It was rare that he called an office meeting, so I figured it was important.

We all showed up and conversated in the main room outside Francis's office, waiting to find out why we were all here.

Francis opened his office door and stepped out. I saw him rubbing his hair frustratedly. He didn't look particularly happy. He found a seat on a table against a wall right outside his office door, "Come on over here everyone," he got our attention and waved us over to gather around him.

I slowly stepped forward, letting others fill in the front rows of the crowd and I situated myself at the back of the crowd.

"As you guys know," He started, animating his hands, "COVID has been rough. But you guys have blown me away. You guys transitioned into working from home amazingly well." He scanned the crowd, making eye contact with me and pointing, "Len, I don't want to hear it."

I started cackling from my spot at the back of the crowd.

Francis continued, "But, the time has come for me to part ways with Cyient. I've thought about it a lot over the last few months. I've even lost sleep over it. It's not a decision I've come to lightly, but I needed to make the announcement and I wanted it to be in person so anyone could ask any questions."

I went from cackling to dead serious in an instant. It was so quiet in there you could hear everyone thinking. We all knew that Francis leaving meant that Chris would be in charge. Chris knew how the business ran, but his people skills were strikingly similar to an adult male baboon, and everyone knew it.

I had questions, but none that I wanted to ask in front of this crowd. I knew I'd get a manufactured PC answer and not the truth. I knew that Francis wouldn't just quit without having something else lined up though, so I knew it was only a matter of time until we found out what that was.

People began to thin out and go home to get their work done, but I stayed and looked for an opportunity talk to Francis.

I knocked on Francis's door after making sure nobody was around.

Joseph was in there talking to him, but he waved me in.

I walked in and gave Joseph a hug before sitting down in one of the open chairs in front of Francis's desk. "What're you guys up to? Super busy?"

"Nah," Joseph said, "We just finished up putting a fire out. You know how that is."

I nodded, "All too well... yes I do, haha." Boy, did I ever? Some days felt like all I did was run around and put out proverbial fires. "I almost put 'Firefighter' as my profession at the dentist the other day." I joked, "So, yoooo..." I prepared to address the elephant in the room, "How's the future looking? I know you wouldn't just quit without a plan and something in the works." I looked at him expectantly.

Francis chuckled nervously, "I mean... okay... look..." he ran the palm of his hand down his face, "I do have something in the works, but it's not ready yet. I'm starting a new business, but everything is still very much a work in progress. It's going to be a very slow process, too, because I have to build it. I can't take any contracts with me. This isn't going to be a thing for a while. I can't even start doing certain things until I've quit this first."

Things were definitely getting interesting at work, to say the least. The future of work seemed very up in the air and uncertain in light of this recent news. I figured it at least made a good opportunity to find out if things get better or worse when Francis leaves. He had his faults, but he had his strengths, too. I honestly didn't know which way it would turn out.

I had noticed how my therapy was helping. Before, I would have likely gotten stuck in an anxiety loop about the uncertainty of the future, but I was able to identify my anxiety and let it co-exist beside me, almost like I was baby-sitting a child. I looked at my options and knew that waiting to see how things turned out wasn't a bad option at all. Perhaps more options would reveal themselves in time, too.

That was new. In the past, I'd let my emotions pressure me into making decisions quickly. I'd search for solutions to a problem until I found two options, and then immediately take the lesser of two evils between the two, thinking I'd solved the problem. I was helplessly unaware that if I just sat still and considered more options, I would eventually find a good one. I was actually learning patience and it felt good to kind of turn around and notice, rather suddenly, that I finally had some patience with myself. It crept up on me.

Only time would tell how this would turn out.

Chapter 19

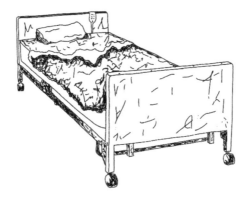

I rolled over in bed and stretched. Warm sunlight filtered through the curtains of my bedroom window. I felt wide awake though, like I had slept for 10 hours. I reached over and tapped the screen of phone. The phone's bright screen flashed "7:22 AM" at me. Not even 7:30 yet? I was up until 2 AM last night, what gives?

I tossed in bed for about 30 minutes in protest, but after a while I knew I wasn't falling back asleep anytime soon. I knew Dad would be up, so I figured I'd give him a call. We hadn't talked in about 6 days anyway.

"Well, hey there, buddy! Didn't expect you to be up so early on a Saturday." Dad answered the phone.

"Heyo Dad!" I responded, "Yeah I don't want to be trust me, haha. My brain just decided it had enough sleep, I guess. How was your week?"

"Ehhh…" He hesitated, "Been better, been worse. Doctor told me it's time to quit smoking. So I haven't had a cigarette in 4 days."

That's a lot more to process than it seems like on the surface level… "Woah, what?" I was trying not to jump to conclusions, but my brain had already landed. "What happened? If the doctors told you it's time quit and you're listening, something serious happened."

Dad started chuckling nervously, "Well damn, yeah you're right. I had a mini stroke earlier this week. I'm fine, though. Doctor said I dodged a bullet, but it's time to take my health seriously."

"Well, that's good," I was genuinely relieved. "I mean, obviously I don't like hearing that you had a stroke, but I'm happy to find out it wasn't a big one. We gotta work on preventing the big one." I said, hoping I was encouraging.

I could hear Dad inhale sharply, "Yeah, we don't want a big one. And because I'm diabetic too, there's even more risk, so I have to tighten up my diet. This sucks, man!" He started laughing.

I started laughing too, "Yeah, it does suck, but we're all going to be so thankful and happy you made the hard choices down the road. We still have to get you guys moved down to Mississippi so we can go camping and fishing and all that." Admittedly, I hated the idea of camping or fishing, but I knew I wanted to build some good memories with Dad. If that meant I had to go camping or fishing to do it, that'd be fine. Donny and Joseph would most likely be coming too if we were going camping, so it would be an awesome time for building good memories.

"Wow... fishing and camping huh?" Dad poked fun at me, "You feeling alright?"

"I mean... yeah, it's not my first choice but it's also not the worst thing in the world. You'd have to teach my nerdy ass a few things I'm sure, but it's not impossible. Who knows, I might actually end up having a good time." I joked.

"Maybe..." Dad agreed playfully.

I continued with my thought, "But we gotta get you guys moved first. Can't really do anything else until we get that first important step done, right?"

"Ehhh, ease up on it, son. It'll happen when it happens. I do want to be down there with you guys, but I've just got a lot of stuff to take care of first. It takes a lot of planning." He responded matter-of-factly.

I winced. I wanted to argue that he was going to put it off until it was too late, but stating that wouldn't do any good. It would just piss him off to call out his choices like that. "Fair enough," I said in defeat, "It just makes me incredibly excited to think about you guys living closer to us. It would make things so much better. I love you, Dad."

After I got off the phone with him, I had to process that. If Dad was starting to go downhill physically, that whole household was going to need help. Dad was the one who made dinners. Maw Maw, his mother, helped him with the cleaning, but for how much longer could she keep that up? She was nearly 80 years old and diabetic. She'd survived breast cancer, twice, but lost both of her breasts. She was a fighter, but not forever.

Maw Maw had lived with them on and off throughout the years. She had recently moved back in with them due to her own declining health.

Nobody in that house would be able to take care of everything forever. It was just a matter of time before they would all need more and more care. I knew that wasn't a sustainable situation, so I felt very pressured to get them moved down here before anything major happened. It would be far easier for us to take care of them if they weren't 800 miles away.

With this changing situation on my mind, I went through another couple weeks of work. I didn't really address anything with Mom or Dad yet, but I was very focused on figuring out a plan to get them down here. Something Dad would see and agree with.

I called them every weekend, but I wouldn't bring up moving. I'd decided to give it a rest until I had something worth bringing to Dad and just work on it in the background until then. But I kept hearing about how worse things were getting up there over time. Maw Maw was diabetic and her feet were black now. She wasn't taking care of herself like the doctors and nurses told her to.

My maternal grandma, Nana, lived with Mom's Sister, Tina, in the same city in Indiana. Nana was in and out of the hospital every other week because she kept falling downstairs. COVID was still a danger, and if either of my grandmas got it, that was game over for them. If Dad got COVID, it would bring the whole house to a halt, and maybe he would survive, but with possible complications for the rest of his life. Fragile...

Mom called me that weekend, per our usual calls.

"Hey Sweetie..." Mom sounded like she was on the verge of crying. Uh oh, this wasn't going to be good...

"Hey Mom, what's up?" I asked, already filled with concern and anxiety.

"It's Nana... she... she passed away last night." She started crying.

I felt numb, but after Alex this just didn't seem that bad. Nana was getting worse and worse. We had been prepared for this for a few months now. She'd lived a long, happy life. That's how life was supposed to work, not like Alex.

I was still sad, but the experience just didn't have any piercing bite to it like Alex's death did. "At least she's not in pain anymore." I tried to reassure Mom.

"Well, there's more." Mom's voice still sounded shaky.

More? I don't want any more... what could possibly...

"I've got you on speakerphone now. Daddy, go ahead." Mom made a dramatic introduction.

I heard dad exhale sharply, "I've got cancer, son."

"Oh wow, um..." Okay, okay, don't panic... Cancer isn't the death sentence it used to be. We've come a long way in cancer treatments, so maybe there's hope. "Well, that's not good, obviously. But we've got options, right? Have you talked to your doctors about any options yet? What do we know about the cancer? When do you start treatment and what does that look like?" I stopped. Breathe, Len. Breathe... Why am I like this?

"I... don't know any of that yet." Dad said slowly, clearly overwhelmed with my questions.

"Okay," I started up again, "Well, I'll plan to come up there so I can help. I work from home, so I can just bring my computer up there and work. We really need to get you down here before you start treatment so you can start it down here. Once you start treatment, it'll be a hundred times more complicated for you to move anywhere." I knew he didn't want to hear that right now, but it needed to be said.

"Yeah, we'll see." He said simply. "It would be nice to have you up here though."

I smiled to myself, "Yeah, it would be, huh?"

So I did. I packed my computer up, told my underlings what was going on and that I would still be available like normal, and headed up. I didn't tell any of my bosses at work because it was probably just easier if they didn't know.

Joseph was able to join me for a couple of weeks, but he eventually had to go back home to work. After a month up there, I realized that it wasn't working for me either. I was too distracted by doing things around the house and spending time with family, so I got almost nothing done. Now I see the problem with working from home and why some of my co-workers still wanted to work in the office through COVID. My situation at home naturally fit itself to working from home, but this situation did exactly the opposite.

I had to call it and go back home. I'd have to go back home and just hope that things stayed good up there as long as possible.

Another couple of months went by like this, and it was agonizing. I'd talk to them every weekend, keeping tabs on the situation up there.

It eventually did get critical, though.

"Hey Mom, what's up?" I answered my phone.

"Hey Sweetie." Her voice sounded shaky again. She knew that was all she had to do to let me know something was wrong.

I took my glasses off and buried my face in one hand, "Oh no... just tell me. What's wrong? Rip the band-aid off."

"Dad, he uh... he, well you know he's diabetic, right?" She asked nervously, opting for the long way around the block.

"Yes of course I know that. Spit it out." I pleaded.

"Well, he woke up this morning feeling fine, but when I tried talking to him, he was talking nonsense. I couldn't understand a word he was saying."

I interjected, "Mom, that's a stroke symptom..."

"I know!" She defended herself, "So I called the doctor and they told me to call an ambulance. So then I called an ambulance and when they showed up-"

I interrupted her, "So where'd they take him? I assume he's in the ER right now?"

"Yeah," She answered, "but I think he had another stroke. Lenny, I'm so scared." Her voice was still shaky and full of emotion.

I managed her back to a state of calm and got off the phone, then worked on calming myself down. Dad had been working up until that incident, and he was sort of forced into taking medical leave at that point.

I knew I was going to need Donny and Joseph's help, so I called them both after I got off the phone with Mom.

"Yo!" Donny answered the phone.

"Sup, Bubba." I greeted back, "Hey listen I've got Joseph on the other line. Let me merge it real quick..." I heard him say 'ok' as I was pressing the button to merge the calls. "Okay, everyone still there?" I asked.

"Yep." That was Joseph's voice.

"Yeah." And that was Donny's, good.

"Aight, so, I'm just gonna put it out there. Dad's in the ER. Mom thinks he had a stroke, but his insulin spiked to some ridiculous amount. I need to head up there so I can help take care of things, and I'm going to need y'all's help." I just put it out there.

Donny snorted in protest, "Man, look, I can't stop working right now. I'll be out there when I can be, but that's all there is to it." He laid the law down.

"Yeah, I'll be able to go with you." Joseph chimed in, "I need some time to figure out my schedule and a couple things, but I'll do what I have to. I wanna be there to help. We can take my truck up."

"Thanks, Bubba, that's most of the logistics handled. I'll help with gas." I paused, fidgeting with my hands nervously for a second, "Donny, what's wrong? Dad's dying and you seem to not really be bothered by it." Was that a mistake?

"Man, look. Mom hasn't done anything but traumatize and ignore me since I was a teenager. I know you don't know all the shit that went down after we moved up to Indiana, but let me tell you it wasn't fuckin' easy. And didn't leave me with the 'warm-n-fuzzies' about Mom or Dad to be frank." Donny was being honest with us, but I felt like Joseph and I were the ones that were going to suffer most from it.

Donny and I's relationship never really had a chance to develop on its own after California. But I was still worried about him and I still wanted to connect with him. I couldn't because he'd always push me away. I appreciated his honesty, but his choices still confused and frustrated me.

"Donny, I get it man. Life ain't peaches. Trust me, that's something that all three of us understand very intimately. I'm not excited about going up and helping. This isn't a vacation for me, but I can't just not do anything at all. I have to go help. Once they're gone, they're gone and all that's left are the memories and regrets. I would rather have more memories than regrets in the end." I'd hoped that maybe my perspective on memories versus regrets would change his mind.

"Whatever man. I can't do it." Donny held his ground.

I started reading the situation as a power struggle between he and I, and didn't really figure that arguing with him would accomplish anything. "Alrighty then. Joseph, we're going to have to think about moving them, too. Their lease is up at the end of this month so they have to move somewhere. We're going to have to help them move down to Tupelo while we're up there." I decided to change the subject.

"Yeah, they do need to be down here so we can take care of them and still keep our lives together. I'll rent one of those big dumpsters. Most of their crap is trash that just needs cleaned up." I could hear Joseph light a cigarette once he was done talking.

"Okay. I've been able to save up some money, so I'll rent the truck once we get everything packed. We'll load it and unload it. Do you know anyone who can drive it for us?" I asked.

"Yeah," Joseph said, "I think I might have someone who would drive for us."

We finished working out the details and planned to head up the following weekend.

By the time we made it up there, we were much needed.

I sat down on the couch next to Dad and Joseph sat on the other side of him. I put my hand on his back and I could feel his spine and ribs protruding from his skin.

"That fffffff... feels..." He thought about the word, "Goober? No... bebber? No... bettered? No..." He could tell that whatever word his brain wanted to produce wasn't right when he heard himself say it.

"Does that feel good?" I asked.

He nodded with a smile of relief, "Yes! Thank you. Damnit man!" He spoke slowly but got all the words right.

Joseph looked at me and we made eye contact. He looked horrified. To be fair, it was sort of horrifying. I'm pretty sure Joseph and I shared a moment of "Oh fuck, this may be way worse than we thought."

I continued to rub Dad's back because it seemed to bring him some comfort. "Well, we're here to help while you're going through treatment. We can't be up here indefinitely though, so we're also going to work on getting you guys moved down to Tupelo. We'll make sure meals get made and people get to their doctor's appointments. We'll also work on packing and throwing trash away and we'll rent a truck and get it all moved. All you gotta worry about is getting better and we'll handle everything else." I stopped rubbing his back long enough to give him a hug.

Dad just nodded silently. A response that I could tell was in defeat.

Joseph and I spent the next two months enduring the hardest time of our lives together. Maw Maw passed away about a week and a half after we first arrived. Her memorial service was in the same funeral home that Alex and Nana had their services at.

We had to learn how to check Dad's blood sugar and how to help him manage diabetes through the meals we made for him. Joseph filled up an entire 40-yard dumpster with ruined furniture, old boxes, old clothes, old everything. I packed and began staging boxes and empty shelves and other large furniture in the front room. Joseph had started working at Francis's new company so he couldn't take any time off from work. He had to do all that and also keep up with work, which he could thankfully do remotely as well.

Donny eventually joined us after Joseph and I had been there for a few weeks. His job required him to be driving a lot, and he had issues with Mom. I couldn't really blame him for feeling the way he did, but because of that Joseph and I had more work to do.

But Dad's health was declining fast. He had started getting up during the middle of the night and getting into random things around the house, so Joseph and I agreed to rotate nights to stay up and watch him. Tonight was my shift to stay up and watch Dad.

"Hey!" Dad grunted, breaking the dead silence in the dark room at 3AM.

I looked over and took a headphone out. He didn't look awake, but he was tossing and turning. I took my other headphone out and set my Nintendo Switch on the table next to me. I slowly and quietly walked over to Dad and sat down on the coffee table in front of his couch, watching him.

"Damnit, Bubba, I told you, you done fucked up now. Get the hell over here." He fidgeted, but his eyes were closed. "Go round everyone up. Yeah, everybody. Meet me at the motor pool." He raised an arm and pointed.

I freaked out a little bit. I swear he was dead asleep, but he was carrying on a full conversation with his old friend "Bubba" and pointing. I guess as long as he doesn't get up, I don't need to respond to anything, but it's still weird.

He calmed back down, and I went back to playing my Switch. 6 AM rolled around and I had to get Dad up for a doctor's appointment.

I walked over and stroked his bald head, "Hey Daddy... It's time to get up. We gotta go get a bath so we can go see the doctor today." He'd only been bald for about a month now, so I still wasn't used to seeing it.

Dad grunted awake. "Hm? Ok... Yep. On my way..." And he immediately turned his head and fell back asleep.

I wanted to cry. I didn't want to wake this poor tired man up, but I didn't have any choice. "Dad, c'mon... we gotta get up now. The doctor's appointment is soon. Let's go get a bath."

I eventually got him up, got him washed in the bathtub, cleaned his bedsore wound, and got him dressed. He didn't say much that day. He probably felt like garbage.

We got to the doctor and they looked at his bed sore. The doctor treated it like a regular checkup and acted like nothing was wrong. Up until now, we believed that Dad's treatment plan stemmed from the goal of Dad surviving.

I pulled Dad's doctor out into the hallway, "So, things aren't looking too good. I'm starting to get really nervous that I'm not equipped to take care of him right now. He just keeps getting worse. Why is he still at home and not in the ER?"

The doctor looked at me, then flipped through his clipboard, "We've got another radiation treatment scheduled in 3 days for him. We'll monitor his health and let you guys know."

I shook my head, "No, I think you misunderstand me. He's hallucinating at night, calling for people who are either dead or not present. Plus I don't know how to take care of his bedsore properly. One person has to stay up during the night with him to make sure he doesn't get into anything dangerous during a weird sleepwalking flashback episode. I'm just not a medical professional and I think he needs to be somewhere where someone can take better care of him. I'm really worried about him." I tried to be as candid as I could be.

The doctor nodded, "We'll keep him here over night if that'll make you feel better?"

If it'll make me feel better? Was he managing my feelings or Dad's health? "It's not about me. It's about Dad's health."

The doctor dropped his clipboard to the side, "Your Dad will be on Chemotherapy for the rest of his life. Chemotherapy isn't pretty."

What the hell did that mean? Was he saying what I thought he was saying? That Dad was as good as dead and there was nothing we could do about it but just watch him suffer through Chemo?

We finished up with the doctor, and they admitted Dad for the night. Donny stayed at the hospital with him and brought him home the next day.

Dad came home with a prescription for Lorazepam though. I knew exactly what that meant. I didn't want to give him the Lorazepam. For some reason, that was what made it seem so final. Even if Dad was alive, he'd be gone after the Lorazepam for sure. No more talks. He'd be out of it until he died. It's how they let people die in comfort.

We sat Dad down in his hospice bed, "So this stuff is gonna help me sleep so I can get better?" Dad asked the nurse.

A sad silence filled the room before the nurse responded, "Yes, Mr. Kester. This is going to help you rest." She answered uneasily. She looked at us, we looked at her. There was no judgment because honestly, nobody knew what to say.

Two soul-grinding days passed. Dad was asleep, periodically talking, but remaining unconscious. I stayed up for two days hoping to catch a few moments with my lucid Father, but on the third day I had to go to sleep. Aunt April, Dad's Sister, had arrived that day. I asked her and my brothers to please wake me up if Dad's condition changed at all.

No sooner than I fell asleep, my brother Joseph came to wake me up.

I came into the front room with one foot firmly planted in reality and the other foot stuck in a dream. It's that weird place you exist when your brain is waking up and trying to determine if you are indeed awake or still dreaming.

I moved my way up to see Dad and I watched him take his last breath.

Chapter 20

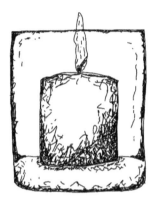

I woke up in the guest bed. Blinking awake, I laid there. Hard to believe Dad was gone now, too. Alex, Nana, Maw Maw, and Dad all died within 2 years of each other. We'd have to take care of Dad's funeral arrangements today. Donny was up here helping, but we still had to finish getting the house packed. We still had about 3 or 4 days of packing left, too. I rolled over and pulled the covers over my head in general protest of life.

As I tried to get back to sleep, I couldn't quit thinking about work. I'd wanted to quit Cyient for a long time. I just didn't care about it anymore. I didn't want to hear about any more missed deadlines or team members who didn't follow directions. I didn't care about the monthly financial reports anymore. I knew I was done with Cyient's circus.

I had slept for nearly 11 hours, so I couldn't fall back asleep. But I really didn't feel like getting out of bed. I reminded myself that I couldn't go home until we were finished, so I got back up and got ready for the day.

I went outside and leaned against Joseph's truck. I pulled a joint out of my pocket and lit it, then pulled out my phone and called my boss.

"Hello?" Mike answered.

"Hey Mike. Just wanted to call and give you an update on things. Dad passed away last night and I quit. I can give you two weeks, but no more than that." I bypassed the small talk and dove right into what I needed to say.

"Well, I'm really sorry to hear about your Dad, but yeah… I kinda figured you'd be quitting soon." I heard his chair creak.

I propped my phone between my shoulder and ear, "Yeah, I honestly don't know why I stayed there as long as I have. This is long overdue."

"I just want to ask you not to tell anyone for a little while. Give me a few and I'll call you back." Mike sounded desperate.

That's weird… but I've already told a couple folks. "Sure." I said, but I didn't care.

A couple hours later, he called me back.

"Hey Len!" He sounded excited.

"Hey Mike. What's up?" I asked plainly.

"Len, I've got some really good news! Really, really good! HR just approved a promotion to section manager for you." Mike proudly announced.

I pinched the bridge of my nose and inhaled slowly, "Mike…" I paused, collecting my thoughts. "Do you remember when I told you that if you waited until I quit to make things right, that it would be too late at that point?"

He huffed "Yeah, yeah, I do, but-"

"Nobody took me seriously." I snapped at him and interrupted him, "Now suddenly everyone feels differently? Don't send that posting to me. I don't want to even see it in my inbox. It's too late, Mike. Tell HR and everyone who asks that I turned down their miraculously well-timed job offer and kindly ask them all to shove a piece of it up their ass. The opportunity to keep me employed there is gone now." I hung up.

I finished my joint and went back inside.

Joseph, Donny, and I had tried to wake Mom up all morning, but she wouldn't move. We knew she was alive because she was snoring. She was out cold though. We tried for probably 20 minutes to wake her up, but she wouldn't even budge. Just more snoring. We suspected that she might have taken something, but we had no clue what and didn't have to time to figure it out. We had to get Dad's funeral arranged and finish packing her things.

We met Aunt April at the funeral home. The same funeral home yet again… By now, just being in that building made me want to crawl out of my own skin. While we were discussing things, Mom's Dad called Donny.

"What'd he want? Everything okay?" I asked Donny.

Donny rubbed his eye, "I guess. Papa just went by the house and saw Mom. He couldn't wake her up either."

All three of us brothers exchanged glances.

"He's on his way here to meet us. He wants to do lunch." Donny added.

We finished making the arrangements there at the funeral home, and we left with Papa to go to lunch.

Papa picked up a fried onion petal and popped it in his mouth. "So, is your Mom okay? I'm really worried about her."

Poor guy. He wasn't ever close enough to Mom to really get to know her. I rubbed my hand across my mouth, "She'll be fine. She probably took something she wasn't supposed to." I shrugged.

"Probably?" Donny's eyebrow was raised so high it nearly popped off his forehead, "You know she took something, it's just a matter of figuring out what it was."

He was right though. We knew she took something.

Joseph made eye contact with me, "Confronting her about this isn't going to be fun."

I looked at Joseph, then to Donny, "Let's just try to enjoy lunch with Papa."

The 4 of us caught up on years of not seeing or knowing each other. He hadn't been involved in my life in any capacity since I was four-years-old. It was nice to catch up with our grandpa, but we eventually had to go back and confront Mom.

We got home and found Mom still sleeping in the same spot. She hadn't moved, but she was still snoring. I poked her and she woke up immediately.

"Eh? Hm?" She said, dazed and confused.

"Welcome back to the land of the living." I huffed and sat down at the kitchen table behind her couch.

"So, how much of what did you take?" Donny said.

"What? I didn't take anything, I'm emotionally exhausted! I just lost my husband!" Mom immediately started crying.

Joseph started going around and collecting all the medicine he could find. I joined him and we made a big pile of our collections on the kitchen table. We had most of Mom and Dad's medicine, but Mom's controlled substances were nowhere to be found. Plus, we couldn't find the Lorazepam.

"Mom," I rubbed my forehead and grimaced, "Where's the lorazepam?"

"The what?" She asked innocently, tears completely turned off now. "I don't know what you're talking about."

"You know exactly what I'm talking about and you're playing dumb. I don't appreciate being treated like that." I scolded her.

"No, I honestly have no clue what you're talking about," She insisted, now starting to cry again.

"You're not going to affect me with your tears. I'm immune to that trick. In fact, it just pisses me off. Lying to me pisses me off even more. You're not doing yourself any favors with me right now." I could feel my patience slipping. I was exhausted and she had slept most of the past 2 months away.

She started stomping, shaking her hands up and down, and yelling, "I'm not lying! I'm not lying! Why won't you believe me?!"

"Are you done with your tantrum yet?" I asked.

"NO!" She shouted, "I'm pissed because you guys think I'm some druggie and won't believe me!"

Just then, Joseph stood up from the couch where she was laying and held up a half-empty tube of lorazepam. He had been searching while we were arguing. That dude was smarter than anyone ever gave him credit for, myself included.

"Uh huh, tell me all about how innocent you are." I pointed at Joseph and walked over to him, grabbing the tube.

Mom immediately tried to grab it from my hands and started shouting. "Give that back! That's mine! It's none of your fucking business what I take!"

I slapped her hand and it surprised her, "I'm not playing this game with you. You have a choice to make right now. I can give you this tube of lorazepam and you can zonk out for as long as it'll let you."

"Give it to me, NOW!" She interrupted and reached for it again.

"Nope, stop it!" I shouted back. I hated doing that, but she wasn't speaking a reasonable language right now, and I had to communicate with her. Once I noticed I had her attention I brought my volume back down to a reasonable level. "I'll give it to you, then I'm leaving and you're never talking to me again in your life. Good fucking luck with moving."

She looked at me in horror.

"Oh, do I have your attention now?" I asked.

She rolled her eyes and huffed.

"Do I have your attention?" I pronounced each syllable painfully slowly.

She nodded.

"Good. If I lose your attention again, I'm out. I'm fucking exhausted. I don't have the energy for games. If you're serious about moving, and you want our help, this Lorazepam is fucking toast. So you tell me right now what you want."

Her face turned so red I thought she was going to pop a blood vessel. I could tell she was thinking about it though.

"And..." I put extra emphasis on the word, "you're going to help us finish packing your shit. There's no excuse for you sleeping all day. If you need a nap, take a short nap. But if you want to move, you're gonna help."

"Why can't you be more understanding?" She said in accusation.

I twitched, "Excuse me?"

"You're so mean!" She tucked her elbows by her side, made fists of her hands, and started crying again.

I stared her in the eye, contemplating whether to say what was on my mind or exercise restraint.

"I just lost my husband and you're taking my medicine and forcing me to work!" She was crying harder than I'd ever seen her cry.

I twitched again. "No doubt this is hard for you. Your children, who just lost their Dad, can't possibly relate. And you know what? We're not taking drugs and passing out on the couch, are we? No. We're continuing to pack your belongings because we're so mean." I was beyond frustrated with her.

Over the next few days, she kept arguing and being difficult with us, so we finished packing everything up and moved it into storage. We had disposed of all the medicine that wasn't prescribed to her, following the hospital's instructions. She was pissed at us for it and wouldn't stop being ugly about it.

We attended Dad's memorial service, but I was emotionally and psychologically checked out for that event. I hated being back at that same cursed funeral home again. As I looked around the attendees, nobody there knew who Dad was. Not really. Dad had no family up in Indiana – it was all Mom's family. And they hated Dad because of the lies Mom would tell her family about him when she wanted to manufacture sympathy to get something from them. This memorial service was for Mom to milk sympathy from all her family, not for the people whose lives had been touched by this man to remember him. I really wanted nothing to do with this sympathy fest.

After the memorial service, we still had a lot to finish up. Mom's lease would be up in just a couple of weeks.

Francis drove up and brought a trailer with him to carry some things. He helped us move Mom's things to the storage facilities in town. We kept anything out of the storage shed that she wanted to keep with her, moved her in with Aunt Tina across town, and went home. She had all of her things packed and staged in a storage facility. She could move wherever she wanted to. She just had to coordinate it and make it happen.

When I got back home, I took a couple weeks to just decompress. I hadn't stopped cooking, packing, and cleaning in two months, and I was exhausted both physically and emotionally. Dad went downhill so fast... I thought he'd beat cancer and we'd have hundreds of weekends left to grill together. In the end, we found out that his lung cancer had metastasized across every organ in his body, including his brain. We had no idea his cancer was that aggressive.

My Dad deserved so much more than he ever got out of life, yet I never heard him complain once. He wasn't a perfect man, but I was proud of who he had become as he grew older. There was a lesson in there I could learn from. Dad was still teaching me lessons after he was gone. Thanks, Dad.

After a couple of weeks of being back home and off work, I was ready to work again. I had already talked with Francis and would be starting at his new company as soon as I was ready. I knew I was ready to work again because I could feel a little bit of boredom set in. Not like before, when Alex died, when I couldn't get a moment to catch my breath. I took my time grieving and mourning Dad, and that made a huge difference this time. It made me wonder, how companies expect people to properly grieve with a mere 3 days?

I had been told I could work from home, so that's the expectation I went into the job with. I also made it clear before I started that work/life balance was hugely important to me. Francis and I had a good understanding of this, and he knew that I would absolutely bust my ass for him in return. It was a proven relationship, if we could get past working from home and working manageable hours.

Telecom engineering is an incredibly complicated and tedious process. There are lots of rules and guidelines that have been built over the last sixty years by the big Telecom companies so that we know how to engineer new infrastructure safely. Each step is built from information learned in the previous step. If you miss something major in the beginning of a project, it can mean that you have to re-do every bit of work you did. That means re-engineering the whole job and re-figuring all the math in a lot of cases.

At Cyient, a lot of our overtime was due to re-work in this fashion. I knew that was a major waste of time and a cause for concern. I had been given a brand new project from a brand new customer by Francis. I did all my research and figured out what we were going to need to do to eliminate re-work on the back end of the job.

I went into the office one day and put a piece of paper in front of Francis after my first week of work there, "Here it is man. That's the list of everything we need to do, in order, to have success with this project you started me on." I was proud. I did my research and was serious about avoiding re-work.

Francis looked it over, "Wait, really? We don't need to do that, c'mon. It'll take so much longer to do it your way, but if we do it this way, we'll save a ton of time." He scratched out a couple things on my list and changed some words around, "There, like that. Do that and we'll be fine."

He completely trashed all that planning I had put into this, but you know, if this is the way he wanted me to do it, who was I to argue with the boss? So I got busy on my project how Francis wanted me to proceed.

Two months down the road, the customer was not happy because the final product didn't have all the right meta-data it needed. I planned to include all that originally, but Francis's plan cut those steps out of my original plan in the interest of saving time. Now we were having to re-do all of the jobs we'd completed over the past two months because of the issue.

"Hey Francis, what's up?" I answered my phone from my office desk at home.

"Hey Len, look we gotta get ahead of this thing. This is a brand new customer. We can't be fucking jobs up right out of the gate like this. I'm gonna have to give this project to Chris to oversee." He genuinely sounded worried.

I scrunched my eyebrows up in thought, "Wait, hold on... by all means, give the project to whomever you want. I'm not going to be upset if someone else wants to run this project, but right at the beginning of this thing, I told you that our Offshore Team was going to need to start the drafting in FROGS so that it would have all the right data in there when we posted it. You told me I was wrong. But if we would have done things the way I originally suggested, we wouldn't have all this re-work right now." I was embarrassed to have to lay it out like that.

"Oh whatever, you didn't know about this back then." Francis protested, "Also, I'm gonna need you to come into the office and work for a few weeks until we get this project back on the rails."

I winced, "What happened to working from home?"

"Well, that's obviously not working, is it?" He retorted.

Suddenly I understood what this was about. Francis honestly didn't even remember what things he cut out of my plan because he most likely didn't even really pay attention to it. He has just been paranoid this whole time about me working from home. When his ideas don't work, he blames it on my working from home being the problem.

"Francis, this whole thing isn't working. Just like Cyient, here we are facing the same problems again." I sighed.

"What?!" He sounded offended, "I addressed the pay issues! I pay way better than Cyient." He defended himself.

I knew I wanted to be careful what I said, "That you did. And I'll give you that one. You pay way more fairly than Cyient did. But it's not about just the pay. The way you run into commitments without fully understanding the scope of the commitment, and then get surprised every time something goes wrong. Then we pay the price for it by working a bunch of stressful overtime to get the project re-worked. Not only that, but you told me that working from home was okay, but it really isn't, is it?"

Francis scoffed, "I'm fine with you working from home, Len, I really am." He insisted, "I just need you to come in for a couple weeks, that's it."

"Francis, I love you man, and I believe you truly intend for me to only be in the office for a couple of weeks. But you know as well as I do that you'll never be comfortable with me working from home. Not only that, but you're putting me under Chris. You know that's a nuclear situation. I just don't have the patience to go through all this stuff again."

"Well, if you don't have the patience for Chris, you might not need to work here. I can't manage your personality conflicts, Len." He snapped defensively at me.

I knew he hated when I ever said anything bad about Chris, but Francis blindly refusing to see Chris's poor behavior didn't leave me feeling warm and fuzzy about my future there. "Well, it pisses me off to hear Chris make fun of gay co-workers, watch him Captain Morgan pose the females, and to watch him treat Jack like garbage. If that's just a 'personality conflict' in your book, then maybe this isn't the place for me, and I should think heavily about quitting." I didn't mean it as a threat, I was being dead serious.

Francis scoffed again, "Oh, that's the hill you're gonna die on?"

"Nope." I said calmly, "The official hill I'm dying on is that this just isn't the right industry for me. I'll work two or three more weeks, but it'll be from home."

"That's okay, we'll be fine. Today can be your last day." Francis said defiantly.

I knew in that moment that I had to find something truly different to do with my life. No job would ever be enough for me because I expected to be treated like a human first, and an employee secondly. The way I expected leaders to act – the way I tried to act to those employees who were under me – was not the way leaders were expected to act anymore. How did someone like Chris still have his job after all the harassing he did around that place?

My wife often used the words, "If I did that where I worked, I'd be fired." She's a manager, so she touches a lot of the same responsibilities as Francis and Chris in her role.

I also knew that 95% of the jobs in America are like this. Where would I go to find my mythological idea of a good leader to get behind who I knew would take care of me if I took care of them? Does such a thing even exist, or was I chasing a complete fantasy? I'm sure good leaders still exist out there, but I have had the worst luck finding one.

Rise or fall, I knew I wanted to do something drastically different with my life. I wanted to do something that I found interesting and satisfying. I wanted to see if I worked with my strengths and fought back against my fears, what could I do with myself?

Chapter 21

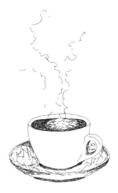

I turned the kitchen sink off, thinking I heard something in the background. I did! I could hear my phone ringer going off from all the way back in the office. I dried my hands off as quickly as I could and sprinted back to the office. I picked up the phone to answer and... I was too late. I just missed the call from my little brother. I immediately called him back.

"Oh, hey!" Joseph answered the phone.

"Hey bud!" I greeted him happily, "Sorry I didn't make it to the phone in time, what's up?"

"Ohhh," He let out a long exhale, "I just finished helping Mom get her trash down to the curb. On my way back to the house now. I was just calling to say hi."

"Epic. I'll take it. How you been since we've been back home?" I asked gently.

"Ehhh..." He hesitated, "Honestly, I've been having a really hard time since Dad passed. But I'm going to see a therapist soon. I've already got the first appointment scheduled."

I knew it wasn't easy for him, but I was really proud to see him handling this much better than I handled Alex.

"I'm glad you're seeking some help man. I think everyone should see a therapist. If nothing else, people would be more aware of mental health and better know how to treat each other."

"Yeah, maybe." He hesitated, "But hey, Mom wasn't doing so great when I was over there."

I closed my eyes and asked the universe for patience, "Oh boy, what's wrong now?"

"She says she's dizzy, and so she sleeps." Joseph sounded bored of it.

I gently shook my head, "She always does this. She pretends to turn over a new leaf, then a few weeks down the line we're back to the strange attention-seeking behaviors. This is so old..." I'd been seeing this behavior pattern in Mom for decades now. I'd still hoped it would change, but that hope had been eroding for a long time now and there wasn't much of it left.

"I dunno, just do me a favor and call and check on her tomorrow for me please?" He asked.

"Of course, Bubba. I'll check on her tomorrow. You know what makes this so hard? The fact that we never really know how much of what she says is truth and how much is lie with her. She has a legitimate medical condition, but she also refuses to take care of herself. How do you deal with the behavioral issues and know when you're running into a legitimate medical issue? You can't take her word for it." I sighed. "I wish it were easier."

I knew that Mom was going to consistently have problems until she got what she wanted. I knew Mom well enough to know that what she wanted was to live with one of us brothers and for us to take care of her full-time like Dad did. She wanted us to cook, clean, and let her sleep every day away.

That life that she wanted, the one that Dad provided for her, wasn't good for Dad or her. It wouldn't be good for us either. There was no way we could let that happen, no matter how hard she struggled against us for it.

I knew this would probably mean multiple hospital visits in our future. That was Mom's thing. She used guilt to get her way. One of her choice tactics throughout the years had been to hospitalize herself somehow. The family would all come running and give her whatever she wanted, and she'd be right as rain until she wanted something else.

I expected to have to push her a bit, but I was also scared because I didn't know where her limitations with epilepsy were. Joseph and I were not at all qualified to handle her as she is, yet here she was.

I was spending my time trying to establish some sort of income. I had a part-time job working for an online barbecue retailer and I had several things I was working on independently. But Mom demanded so much of my attention.

I knocked on Mom's door and looked over to Liz, then Joseph, "What has she done now?" I rubbed my forehead.

A few moments later, Mom stumbled to the door and unlocked it, stumbling back toward the living room. I walked in and followed her into the living room. She was scraping pills out of the cushion of her chair.

Joseph grabbed the wad of medicine from her, "Mom, why were you digging wet, mushed up pills out of the chair?"

She looked up at Joseph with disgusted confusion, "Huh? These are cookies." She held up her other hand with more pills in it.

Joseph grabbed the other pills from her, "Jesus, Mom, what are these? What are you doing?"

Mom looked at Joseph with confusion.

I reached a hand toward Joseph, "Can I see those?"

He handed them to me and walked off, shaking his head.

I took them and inspected them, "Well, whatever these were, there's no telling what it is now. These are ruined." The first handful was wadded into a single clump of soggy powder. It had to have been 4-5 pills worth of material. I wondered if she was OD'ing on something to trigger her next hospital visit. I had no clue what was going on and I was scared, so we called an ambulance.

Mom spent the next 3 days in the hospital.

When she got out, we found out that she almost OD'd on one of her meds. I'm sure it was one of her sleep cocktail meds, but she wouldn't tell us which one it was. Whatever it was, she was out of her mind on it.

We took her home and Liz, Joseph, and I had a long conversation with her.

"Mom, you've got to take care of yourself. How many hospital visits is it now? 5? 6? I've lost track already." I looked at Mom dead in her eye, but she looked away.

"I can't take care of myself!" She protested and started crying.

I winced, "Yes, you can. You just refuse to. You've refused to for so long now

that it's not going to be easy at all. But you have to. That's the only option."
I paused, contemplating my next words carefully, "Look, the doctor and the
social worker at the hospital told me you're one-hundred percent fine and able
to take care of yourself medically. You don't have a legitimate excuse not to
take care of yourself. I know we fight because you want us to take care of you
and we want you to take care of yourself."

She scoffed sarcastically, "Yeah we sure do."

So she acknowledges it... "Yeah, so if you'd spend less energy fighting with
us and more energy taking care of yourself, life would be better for everyone
standing in this room right now." I looked around to Joseph and Liz, then back
to Mom. "The choice is yours, but you're the only one who's going to suffer if
you choose to not take care of yourself."

That was so hard telling her this. These are things a parent should teach a
child, not the other way around.

Mom put her head in her hands and started sobbing. She looked
picturesque. I wondered if she did that on purpose. I also wondered if anything
from this conversation would stick. We had a conversation just like this every
time she got out of the hospital.

We made sure she had what she needed and left. On our way back home,
we talked about it.

Joseph glanced at me, momentarily taking his eyes off the road, "Man, I
need help."

I tilted my head in concern, "What's wrong, Bubba?

He adjusted his grip on the steering wheel, "Just with Mom. She's too
much. She always wants me to come take her trash out and do this little thing
or that little thing. It's constant."

I sighed, "You know how I've been trying to get Donny to forgive Mom for
like, years now?"

He nodded.

"Well, after Mom took that Lorazepam, it fucked all that up. Donny's been
telling me for years that she'll never change, and he's right. He distanced
himself from her for his own sanity. I was mad because by choosing not to
help Mom, he was also making things harder for us without his help. It hurt
because it felt like it was me that Donny wasn't wanting to help."

Joseph squinted, "Okay…" I knew he was looking for the purpose in what I was saying.

"Point is, now I'm in his position and you're in my position and I have a better understanding of both sides now. It's hard man. It's really hard. Because Mom isn't going to change until she chooses to. But she's going to continue to milk as much help from others as she can. That's who she is. She plays these emotional games with people, man. She needs to be taking her own trash out and doing things on her own. She'll do as little as we let her get away with."

Joseph thought for a moment, toying the steering wheel idly, "I get that, but I can't just tell her no…"

"She's going to want to continue doing the same things she's always done until we force her to find a different way to get what she wants. It's not gonna be easy, but even the case worker at the hospital said it sounded like Mom needed some tough love from us right now." I reached across the cab of his truck and put my hand on his shoulder.

Joseph sighed. I knew he hated it as much as I did.

Liz spoke up from the back seat of the truck, "You have a responsibility to yourself before you do to anyone, parents included. You have your whole life ahead of you. She can learn, and I'm sure she will in time, we just have to be strong and set a good example for her."

"You're not wrong about that…" Joseph agreed.

Joseph dropped Liz and I off at home and we settled in for the night.

I went to bed at around 10 PM with Liz, but it was 1 AM and I still couldn't sleep, so I decided to get back up. I realized I hadn't eaten anything in a couple of days, so I made some oatmeal and continued working on a project at my computer.

The sun came up and so did Liz. She got ready for work, and I made some coffee for her. I decided to have a cup, too, because how can you make coffee and not have a cup? I'm not a religious man, but that's heresy.

Liz rushed through the kitchen, drying her hair after her shower. "Another bad night?"

I leaned against the island counter in the kitchen, "Yeah, but it's fine. This is why I have a part-time job and not a full-time job. Working from home helps a lot, too." I raised my voice enough so that she could hear me from the bedroom where she hurried to.

"I'm sorry," her voice echoed from the bedroom, "You think it's a depression or an anxiety thing?"

I swallowed a sip of perfect coffee, "Probably a little bit of both, if I had to guess? But I'm not too worried about it."

Liz walked into the kitchen looking ready for work.

I pointed to the counter in front of the coffee pot, "I made you a cup of coffee over there."

"Oooooooohhh..." She lit up and walked over to the cup, securing it with both hands. "Thank you!" She sipped.

I smiled, "Of course! You're awesome and I love you."

Off to work she went. I let Moby outside on his lead and went back to my PC. I knew I was feeling depressed, so I allowed myself the space I needed to exist with it and used my projects as a way to keep busy with something while depression hung around and did its thing.

It was Friday, so I was excited about game night tonight. We've had our ups and downs as friends, but we're still here doing our Friday night thing every week. The ups and downs we've gone through together only strengthened the bond we've created.

"WHO DA FUCK?" I heard Thomas greet me as I entered the Discord channel. Thomas was definitely the life of our party.

"Yooooooooooo!" I howled in greeting.

"Len, we in here bullying bots. Where you at?" Luci invited me to come play Overwatch 2 with them.

"Oh, I'm updating now!" I replied excitedly, rubbing my hands together and watching the download progress bar fill up quickly.

"Oh shit, incoming! My ult!" Ingram said.

"Ahhhhh!" Thomas and Luci shouted battle cries as the enemy team of AI bots charged the capture point they were defending.

"Team Kill!" JP triumphantly shouted. "Great job, they showed up out of nowhere!"

"Aight, I'm in. Put me in, coach! Let me at 'em!" I announced and accepted the party invite that followed. We were goofballs no matter what we were playing. That's what made it great. No matter what happened during the week, we knew what to expect out of Friday night and knew we could unwind comfortably with each other.

After a few matches, the conversation shifted to more serious matters.

"Yeah, Mom had another hospital visit this week. She just got back home... uh... yesterday? Day before? I dunno, I haven't been to sleep in almost 40 hours, so time is a lil weird, but she's back home now in any case. She keeps letting herself get into trouble medically to cry for attention. I'm kinda sick of giving her attention." I divulged in my friends.

"I'm sorry man, I wish I could fix things for you." I could hear the empathy coming out of JP's voice.

"You're a sweetheart, man. I appreciate you, but it's just a thing in life that I gotta deal with. I love her, but I can't force her to take care of herself." I sighed.

We eventually wrapped it up for the night and I slept like a baby for the following 10 hours. Sleepless nights happen completely on their own. Sometimes I can go months without having sleep problems, and then have problems sleeping for a full week. Same thing with eating. I can go months with a normal diet, but then just not eat anything at all for 3 or 4 days before I get hungry again.

I've also made some good friends out of my larger gaming community. Some of the friends I have whom I only talk to across Discord or video games are among the best friends I have. Some of these relationships seemed more real and beneficial than some of the relationships I'd built with coworkers and fringe people in my life.

No doubt, the fringe people in my life simply thought I'd lost my mind and become hermit. But in truth, I had trimmed the fat from my life. I couldn't worry about how it looked to anyone else. I had to worry about making it work for me. Sure, it was a bit hermit-ish, but I had a full network of friends and being at home works for me. It wouldn't work for everyone. In fact, it wouldn't work for Liz. But it works for me.

My life had been trimmed down from the chaotic nonsense it was. Life was calmer and I could think and focus. No more weekly drinking parties, and no more emotional over-extending.

I'm not sure what "healthy" looks like, but life had become better even if depression and anxiety hadn't completely disappeared. They're still a big part of the equation, but therapy gave me the tools I needed to manage them.

I've had to change my lifestyle to fit it as well. I can't make the commitment that companies are demanding these days, so I explore other avenues independently now.

Liz is really my secret weapon, though. She has been the best battle buddy ever. After we separated and got back together, our relationship was set in concrete. And she's been right behind me the whole way. The silent rock that I reach out to for stability when I stumble. And I do stumble.

I woke up after my 10 hours of sweet sleep. I rolled around in bed and looked at my phone. Alex was still gone. Dad was still gone. Mom still worried me. I still had the sexual trauma. I pulled one foot at a time out from under the blankets and planted them on floor. I rub my eyes to get the eye crusties out, and I go take my shower for the day.

And so, life goes on. Day by day. Cup of coffee by cup of coffee.

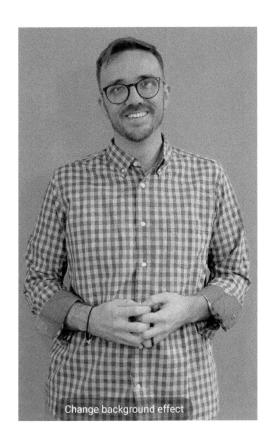

Change background effect

Len Kester is a teacher and a writer who believes in the simple and subtle power of choice. Len has taught Jr. High and High School English and also helped engineer over 5 million feet of fiber optic telecommunications lines for rural communities with the goal of impacting others for the greatest positive effect. His debut memoir is a reflection of his desire to contribute to the overall conversation on mental health for destigmatizing & normalizing further discussions about it. You can find Len at www.lenkester.com.

Milton Keynes UK
Ingram Content Group UK Ltd.
UKHW020704231023
431165UK00016B/759